Pop's Garden Gift
The Journal of a Garden, its Seasons, and a Man

By

Richard Clay Forbes

Westview Publishing Co., Inc., Nashville, Tennessee

© 2008 by Richard Forbes.

All Rights Reserved. No portion of this book may be reproduced in any fashion, either mechanically or electronically, without the express written permission of the author. Short excerpts may be used with the permission of the author or the publisher for the purposes of media reviews.

First Edition, March 2008

Printed in the United States of America on acid-free paper.

ISBN 1-933912-85-5

Edited by Lou Hughes

Cover design by Landon Earps

Typography by Mary Catharine Nelson

Prepress by Westview Book Publishing, Inc.

WESTVIEW PUBLISHING CO., INC.
P.O. Box 210183
Nashville, Tennessee 37221
www.westviewpublishing.com

Dedication

This book is dedicated to my wife Ann, her brothers, and the grandchildren and great grandchildren of James Alton Young (Pop) and Jane Hardwick Young (Grandma). The garden on Wilhugh Place in Nashville, Tennessee has either been etched into their memories, or related to them in storied fashion.

Pop and Grandma's children, and their families:

Ann Young Forbes and husband Rich
Children: Mariah Forbes Daly and husband Mike, Holly Forbes Girdler and husband Josh, Chris Forbes, Jim Forbes.
Grandchildren: Madden Daly, Jane Ann Girdler, Joshua Girdler.

Carol Denise Young

David Young and wife Susanne
Children: Warner Young, Janie Young.

Don Young and wife Christine
Children: Jonathon Young and wife Heather, Ben Young, Chase Young and wife Kristen, Chelsea Young, Jennifer Reinhardt, Amie Reinhardt, Bobby Reinhardt.
Grandchildren: Alyssa Young, Ethan Young.

Joe Young and wife Beckye
Children: Benjamin Young, Daniel Young, Hannah Young, Jacob Young.

Richard Clay Forbes

Contents

Preface .... *vii*
Introduction *3*
The Withering *5*
Fallow *9*
Preparing the Garden for Winter *11*
Winter Planning *17*
Planting the Greenhouse *21*
The Quickening *27*
Planting Time *43*
Growing In the Sun While *59*
Clouds Gather *59*
First Harvest *79*
Final Harvest *85*
Planting Cotton *99*
James Alton Young (Pop) *101*

Pop's Garden Gift

Preface

My First Days with Pop and the Garden

Before there was a Grandma or Pop, there was Mr. and Mrs. Young. As for me, I was a bearded young man fresh from Virginia and the Virginia Military Institute who burst into their lives through my involvement with their lovely daughter Ann.

The year was 1974 and Ann and I were attending college, she was a new freshman and I was a senior. We started dating and fell in love. Other than going to class, and occasionally sleeping, we were always together.

It didn't take long for Ann's mother, Mrs. Young, to hear that there was a boy at school and things were getting pretty serious. So, she and Mrs. Hardwick (Ann's Grandmother) decided it was time to drive to McKenzie, Tennessee and meet this fellow. The plan was for them to spend the day with Ann and they asked her if I would have lunch with them. In reality, the whole trip was to find out who this young man was.

Lunch went well and I absolutely loved the two of them. Apparently they thought I was alright as well because the next weekend Ann's father showed up to check this out for himself. He stepped out of his car, took one look at me and said "Lost your razor?" Being quick witted as I am, I chose the wrong moment to joke around. I said "Well Mr. Young, you know we are having an energy crisis and this is my attempt to help Gillette make production." My attempt at humor was greeted with a stern stare and he was off to see the dorm mother.

Despite a glowing recommendation from the dorm mother, I was still totally unacceptable to Mr. Young. Each time I would visit the Young's, Mrs. Young would greet me warmly while Mr.

Young wouldn't even speak to me. I guess he thought that if he ignored me I would go away.

At Christmas I proposed to Ann and she accepted. We sat down with her parents and whenever Mr. Young would want to say something to me he would look right at Ann and ask the question. She would then look at me and I would answer. Finally he agreed to the marriage if we would wait for a year. Near as I could tell he thought that this would give him time to run me off.

Ann had three brothers, Don, David, and Joe. Her brother David took pity on me and devised a plan that he thought would help. He asked me if I would consider staying with them that summer and work with Don and him mowing grass. His theory was that Mr. Young would get to know me and maybe even learn to like me.... A little. I agreed and the plan was implemented.

Summer came and I moved into the Young's basement with David and Joe Young. We mowed grass and had a great time. Meal time was a bit strained. Mr. Young would never say a word to me. If he needed to ask me a question at the dinner table he would direct it to Ann and I would respond. It was as if I were a ghost.

Weeks went by and just as I thought that this wasn't going to work, Mr. Young announced that he needed someone to help him shovel horse manure from a local barn. He wanted this for his garden. He asked each of his sons and in turn each informed him that he was busy. Jumping at the opportunity I said that I would help.

The weekend came and we climbed into the pickup truck to go to the farm. It was a quiet ride with not one word spoken. By the time we arrived I had decided that for every shovel of manure that Mr. Young put into that truck, I would put two. We worked feverishly through the morning. Then the miracle happened, Mr. Young spoke to me! I answered, and he spoke again!

After our bond was forged with shovels and manure, we had a great relationship. Maybe all of those psychologists are right... you do have to work at a relationship. Regardless, it has been over thirty years since that day and without fail, he always treated me like a son.

I often remind Ann that I had to shovel manure for her, but that she was worth every shovel full. She hates the analogy, but appreciates the work I did with that shovel. We have been happily married for over thirty one years.

The years passed by and Grandchildren came to the Young family. Mr. and Mrs. Young became Pop and Grandma. Their new titles of endearment were adopted by all. The garden, that had helped me win Mr. Young's approval, thrived. I had no clue that one day this garden, that had already given me a wife, would reach out to me once again

Pop's Garden Gift

Pop's Garden Gift

Pop's Garden Gift

Introduction

This is the story of a gardener, his apprentice, and the last crop he made. It is a tale of one man and his son-in-law, but is a story shared by many gardeners and their children.

In 1953 a young gardener and his wife bought a parcel of land on Wilhugh Place in Nashville Tennessee and built a home. They raised a family and made a garden there, each with the same loving care. Every year the garden became an easel on which the gardener painted a masterpiece for his family. They lived, loved, and prayed in the house by the garden, and it nourished them.

After many years, the gardener became aged, and his ailments made it impossible for him to tend his garden. A son-in-law stepped forward and became the apprentice who would receive the knowledge of gardening, and as it turned out, more than he could ever have imagined. This is his story of their garden together

Pop's Garden Gift

The Withering

I rode back and forth over the yard on a John Deere lawn tractor, lost in the calm of a perfect summer day. Contrary to my many complaints regarding yard work, I actually enjoyed the quasi mindless task. It gave me an escape from the hectic pace of life, allowing my mind to wander beyond the tedium to more poetic pursuits.

On this day I was mowing my in-laws' yard. They have reached an age where the simple pleasure of mowing grass has become impossible. I volunteered to maintain the yard out of love for these two parents. They took me into their lives and family more than thirty years previous, and I feel fortunate to be able to help. It is more than worth the time away from my wife Ann and the kids.

Grandma, my mother-in-law, is a gentle quiet woman who lives her life with the bible as her guide. She hugs me when I arrive for a visit, and again when leaving. She has done this every time she has seen me for over thirty years. She is like my own mother.

In his younger years my father-in-law, Pop, was a hard working man with a keen mind who ran his family with authority. However, age has finally caught him and his body is betraying his once determined manner. The bruises and cuts on his arms are evidence of frequent falls; a constant reminder of his ever progressing congestive heart failure.

The mower bags were approaching full so I turned the tractor towards the backyard and a large pile of leaves and clippings behind the garden. Honeybees flew past me in the sweet breeze as I passed their hives alongside the hedgerow. I didn't notice that I had company in the garden.

I turned the mower blades off and followed a path worn down along the back fence between the shrubs, which Pop had grown from cuttings, and the garden proper. It wasn't until I made the final turn in front of the leaf pile that I noticed him. He was sitting in a folding chair strategically placed at the end of a row of tomatoes. His walker was close by his side.

Pop was staring intently down the rows of tomatoes when I walked up beside him. "Have you ever seen such crooked stakes?' he asked. I looked down the rows and thought that they looked pretty straight to me. "I can't complain though, I appreciate Bill staking them for me" he continued. I laughed and pretended to agree with him.

Bill Hughes is married to Pop's sister Ruby. The two of them have been trying to make the garden presentable in what might be the last year Pop would see it. Whenever they have spare time they weed, water, stake, and tie tomato plants. The previous year Ruby had wept when she saw how overgrown his garden had become. He had fallen ill shortly after the spring planting and became unable to care for it.

"I should never have started a garden this year" he sighed. I knew this wasn't how he felt. Pop was a gardener who took great pride in what he grew and in the beauty of his garden. The lack of attention, as evidenced by the miniature tomatoes clinging to the vines, was just another reminder of his failing health.

Don, Pop's oldest son, knew that his father loved this garden when he planted tomatoes, beans, corn, peppers, and okra earlier in the spring. The ingredient he couldn't give was care. Don planted out of love, but he traveled extensively and overlooked the pride that Pop took in his garden. Watching plants come out of the ground and then wither or be choked by weeds was worse than torture to him.

"Do you think this will be my last garden?" he asked me, never diverting his gaze from the withering plants. I responded, "No Pop, it will look better next year." I knew that he might be right, but I couldn't bring myself to acknowledge it. My eyes welled. So I responded "We had a cool spring and very little rain this year." I was making excuses for the lack of attention that, had he been healthy, Pop would have lavished on this garden.

The summer passed into fall as I continued to regularly mow the lawn. His trips to the garden became less frequent. The garden died and was overtaken by weeds. Pop became frailer with the passing season. They were failing together; Pop and this garden he so treasured.

Pop's Garden Gift

Fallow

The leaves began to fall and blow in the autumn winds. I now rode the tractor to mulch and suck them from Pop's lawn. Making my trips to the compost pile at the back of the garden to dump leaves now seemed futile. The garden that had needed them in prior years was covered in tall weeds and seemed to cry with a ghostly moan as the wind blew over it. I shivered on the tractor.

Garden dreams began to haunt me. The sight of Pop sitting at the end of a withering row of tomatoes weighed heavy on my heart. The look of despair on his face as he surveyed the weeds towering over the pepper plants ate at me. Would this be the last image I would have of this once proud gardener?

I toyed with the idea of making Pop's garden myself, but I knew that my gardening skills were more than limited. Would I be the one he would look at when the plants were failing? I could hardly endure that thought. What about the weather, would my prayers be answered for rain and sunshine? Would God smile on my attempt to show this man I cared so much for one last garden?

I thought about Pop's past trips to Doctor Thomas Frist Sr., and Doctor Karl Van Devender's offices. He would carry a grocery bag full of tomatoes and beam as he handed it to them. He was giving a part of himself, a gift as precious as any he had. Although Pop was blessed with having two exceptional physicians, the aging Doctor Frist understood this best and would call him at home to ask if he had any more tomatoes. Pop would select his best and take them to Dr. Frist's home where they would sit for hours and talk. Their friendship grew, yet Pop always referred to him as Doctor Frist out of respect for his age.

This was a man who had saved Pop's life on more than one occasion.

There was also the pride he had for his daughter Ann as she canned Chili Sauce (similar to chow-chow) from the proceeds of his garden. The recipe had belonged to Grandma's mother and is a family treasure. I couldn't tell if Pop was more pleased that she was maintaining a family tradition or allowing him to once again become the provider. Either way, the joy and pride was evident in his smile and demeanor.

Finally I made a decision. I called my wife on her cell phone to gain her support. "Ann, I want to make Pop's garden next year" there was silence on the other end. "Are you there?" I asked at last. Her sobbing voice came back to me, "That would be great. Do you think he will be alive next year?" It hurt inside when I responded "sure he will", but my voice betrayed the doubt. I wondered if I had waited too long to intercede in the garden?

I told her that if I took on this task it would mean time away from home. I wouldn't do it unless I could give the garden the same care that Pop would expect. Ann agreed again, she loved her father too much, and knew what this would mean to him. She volunteered to help me when I needed her. I wondered again if I had waited too long to make this decision. "Let me ask Pop" I said.

Preparing the Garden for Winter

Friday, October 6, 2006

Pop is having company tomorrow; his sister Ruby has arranged for his surviving brother and sisters to meet at his house for a reunion and lunch. Due to Pop's poor health, the family wants to get together for a visit.

I took a vacation day today so that I could get Pop's yard mowed, his driveway and patio swept, and his garden cleared of weeds, and tilled.

I arrived at 9:00 A.M. to begin my day's work. Pop and Grandma had gone to the grocery so I took my blower and blew the oak leaves and acorns off the driveway. I try to do this often so that they won't fall when going to the mailbox.

After clearing the driveway and patio, I trimmed the yard with a push mower. Just as I was finishing the trimming, Pop and Grandma came home from the grocery. They were surprised to see me, and I helped them bring in the groceries. Pop was tired and needed a rest in his recliner.

I returned to my duties, backed the yard tractor off the carport, and started mowing the yard. My plan was to mow the yard then, unbeknownst to Pop, start working on the garden.

After making my final pass over the backyard, I made my trip to the leaf pile behind the garden and shut the tractor off.

It was a cool day with a projected high of seventy degrees. I started untying the tomato plants from their stakes. This was a slow process because the weeds had grown up around them and

Pop's Garden Gift

the strings were plentiful and tied in knots. I had completed three of the twenty four plants when Pop appeared at the corner of the garden, supported by his walker.

I said "Hey Pop" and he replied, "I didn't hear your mower and thought something might be wrong." I told him no, that I was done with the yard and wanted to clean up his garden. I took the opportunity and said, "Pop there's something I want to ask you" to which he responded "what's that Rich?"

I continued, "I don't want to jump in here if Don wants to do this again next year, but if you will let me, I would like to do your garden in the spring." I expected him to think about this for a while, but he answered right away "it's yours!" I assured him that I would do a good job and that with his knowledge and my labor the garden would return to its past splendor. He was more than pleased. I could see the sparkle of his eyes.

"While you're up here" I said, "show me how to use the tiller." He smiled and proceeded to instruct me on the nuances of his old Troy Bilt tiller. He stood at the end of the garden and gave me tips as I made several passes. Soon I was on my own.

After working about a quarter of the garden, I looked up to see him whacking weeds with a stick. It just wasn't his nature to stand idly by while someone else worked. I smiled to myself and continued on until I reached the rows of weed infested tomatoes where I shut the tiller off and went back to untying strings.

Pop stayed with me a while longer, showing me which tomato poles were worn out, and helping me complain about the knots, before shuffling back to the house for a rest.

I finished my job with the strings and pulled and stacked the poles by the fence as Pop had instructed. I then mowed the weeds that remained and tilled the vacant rows that once contained tomatoes.

Pop thought that the weeds had killed two long rows of strawberries he had planted, but after close inspection, I found that most could be salvaged. I took the tiller and ran back and forth down the rows getting as close to the strawberries as I could get without hitting them.

My strategy worked and soon I had two nice rows of strawberries. I needed to hand weed the rows and straw them, but they would be saved.

With the yard looking good and the garden tilled (with the exception of the strawberries) I put up my tools and headed to the house. Pop was sitting in the porch swing on the patio and kept telling me how nice everything looked. I knew that it meant a lot to him, but my reward was even greater... his pleasure and approval.

We talked a bit about crabgrass and Bermuda, before the subject of fertilizer came up. I told him that I had been thinking of sending a soil sample to the University of Tennessee Soil Testing Lab before buying fertilizer. He thought for a moment before saying "that's a good idea." He was allowing his young apprentice to try something new.

I left for home at 6:30 P.M. tired, but pleased with a good day's work.

<u>Saturday, October 7, 2006</u>

Today Pop was visited by his brother Earl, and sisters Ruby, Geraldine, and Eunice. It was a good visit and the yard and garden looked great.

I took advantage of being back at Pop and Grandma's by filling two plastic Zip-Loc bags with soil from the garden. I will take them to the lab for testing next week. This should tell us what fertilizer and lime mix we will need to add and till in.

Tuesday, October 10, 2006

I took the soil sample to the Soil Testing Lab today. They were incredibly nice and said that my testing would be done the next day. I was a bit confused by the number of tests available, but the lady working in the lab said that the basic test would give me everything I needed to know regarding fertilizer and lime.

I called Pop and filled him in on the trip to the lab. He said that he thought we might need lime because he had been composting with leaves and that they took the lime out of the soil. Something tells me that he will be proven right!

Friday, October 13, 2006

The soil sample results arrived in the mail today. I was more than surprised to see that the soil Ph was 6.9. This is just a paltry .1 below neutral. The recommendation was not to add lime at this time. As for the fertilizer; all levels were in the high category. No fertilizer was needed either! I guess that it shouldn't have shocked me when I found that Pop's garden was perfect.

I called him and read the results over the phone. He pretended to be surprised that the garden didn't need anything. I'll bet that he was smiling on the other end of the line. The old master was still in control!

Pop's Garden Layout

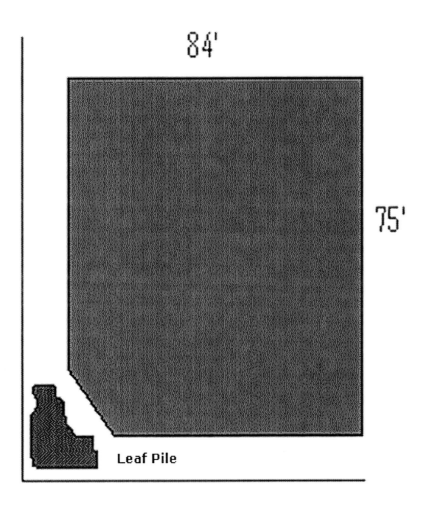

Pop's Garden Gift

Winter Planning

Genesis 1:29: And God said, Behold, I have given you every herb bearing seed, which is upon the face of all the earth, and every tree yielding seed; to you it shall be for meat.

Friday, January 5, 2007

After a long day at the office, I walked slowly into the kitchen. I was glad that the weekend had finally arrived and felt drained by the grey of winter and a week of dark early mornings.

Ann was busy at the kitchen counter but she hadn't started preparing dinner yet. I greeted her with my normal "Hey Baby!" and suggested that we go out for dinner somewhere. The suggestion was met with enthusiasm. Ann was equally ready to start her weekend with a bit of pampering (beginning with no cooking).

As we put on casual clothes in preparation for an evening out, Ann mentioned that Pop had selected seeds from his garden catalogs and wanted to talk to me about them. I was somewhat surprised, given that I had ordered several catalogs and only one had arrived. Ann went on to tell me that Pop had a twenty five dollar coupon and he wanted to use it before the expiration date. I smiled and chuckled to myself. Once again Pop was way ahead of me. He was planning the garden.

I was also amused at the use of a discount coupon. Given the amount of work that goes into a garden, the discount seemed trivial, but over time I had come to realize that saving money was as big a part of the ritual as the sharing of the garden's bounty. There is a certain sense of accomplishment in saving money.

Wednesday, January 10, 2007

I left my office promptly at 11:00 A.M. for lunch with Pop and to go over the plan for the garden. The drive to his house took a short fifteen minutes and I thought about my choices of vegetables as I drove.

I walked into the house to find Pop on the phone. I nodded hello and made my way into the kitchen. Grandma was almost always there and today she was shuffling about cleaning as I said "hello Mrs. Young!" There was almost an excitement in her voice when she greeted me. She is always glad when family comes by; it breaks the monotony of quiet days alone. As Grandma and I made small talk about family and whether I had eaten lunch yet, Pop called from the den, "You want to talk garden Rich?'

I knew that Pop had selected some seeds, but what I didn't realize was that he had planned the structure of the garden right down to how many rows of each type vegetable we would plant, where the cantaloupe and watermelon hills would be, and which plants we could wait until spring to purchase.

My decision to take on the garden was already bearing fruit. I hadn't seen Pop this excited in quite some time. It warmed me to see him enjoying something this much. He had a focus again and this was more than important for Pop.

The garden had become the glue that would bind us together at a very personal level, one that I wouldn't fully understand until much later. The garden was Pop, and Pop was the garden. Now he was letting me enter this very important part of his life.

We went through the list of plants that he had selected. The quantity was almost scary for a novice like me, but I was reassured that we could handle it.

From the Henry Fields catalog he had selected:

- Beefmaster Tomatoes
- Better Boy Tomatoes
- Big Beef Tomatoes
- Beefsteak Tomatoes
- Delicious Tomatoes
- Brandywine Tomatoes
- Henry Fields Pepper Sweet Peppers
- Sweet beauty Cantaloupes
- Athena Hybrid Cantaloupes
- Sweet Gem Hybrid Cantaloupes
- Sparkle Sup Cantaloupes
- Jewel Cantaloupes
- Eversweet Watermelons

From the Parks Seed catalog came:

- Vertical stakes and accompanying name tags
- Ambrosia Cantaloupes
- Yellow Crook Neck Squash
- Cool Breeze Hybrid Cucumbers.

We discussed the beans, and I was assigned the task of ordering them. I had selected two varieties of bush beans. We would plant a row of each. Pop suggested that the corn and okra be purchased locally in the spring. I knew that my time would be precious once the gardening began.

With the garden plants and design agreed upon, we went to the kitchen table to have lunch. Grandma wasn't going to let me go back to work without eating. I knew better than to refuse.

Friday, February 9, 2007

The phone rang this morning and it was Pop. "The seeds came in," he announced. There was excitement in his voice. "We will need to get some potting soil and some flats (low sided trays) to start them in. If we can't find enough flats, we can start the tomatoes in plastic cups with a hole in the bottom." He was talking quickly as his mind went through the steps we would need to follow.

I asked him how much time we had before we needed to plant the starter plants, and he replied, "six weeks before we set them." He added, "I get confused with the planting date these days." This is one thing that I knew. Through the years, I have heard Pop say over and over again that you can plant in Nashville after the tax man comes, or in other words, after April 15th.

I told him that I would get the flats, a bag of fertilizer, and potting soil. Garden time is close at hand.

Planting the Greenhouse

When you walk out the back door of Pop's house, you immediately see the greenhouse. It is a half arch shaped structure that attaches to the house just under the eave and extends out into the yard ten feet. The frame is made of aluminum and supports clear plexi-glass panels.

This is where every garden begins and miracles are realized. Trays of seeds will fill the spaces between patio plants stored there for the winter. By planting time the greenhouse will be full of green plants waiting to be transplanted into the garden, or moved onto the patio.

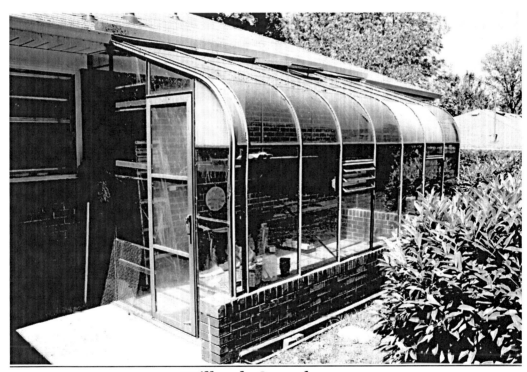

Wilhugh Greenhouse

Pop's Garden Gift

Saturday, March 10, 2007

It was a beautiful Saturday morning that teases you with the arrival of an early spring. The temperature was predicted to reach the mid seventies and made indoor chores seem much less attractive. After a split second of thought, I decided to plant the seeds that Pop had bought and place them in the greenhouse to germinate.

On the ride over to his house I thought about the lack of phone calls I had received regarding the seeds. Typically Pop would call and remind me of jobs that needed to be done around his house. His memory had started failing and often I would receive two or three phone calls in a single day, all about the same subject. He would often forget that he had already called.

I stopped by the garden center on the way and picked up a fifty pound bag of seed starting soil, peat pots, and plastic trays to set them in. I wanted to be ready to plant seeds the moment I arrived. I had material for 182 plants. I was ready!

I walked into Pop and Grandma's house and announced my arrival. The house was quiet and no greeting was returned. As I rounded the corner into the dining room I could see them through the window, sitting in the swing on the patio. They were enjoying the warmth and sunshine. It warmed me to see them sitting side by side like a couple of young lovers.

I opened the back door and loudly announced "Good Morning!" The response from them was immediate. They love company and were excited that I was there. I told Pop that I was ready to plant seeds, and his response puzzled me. He said "we can do that today, but we have plenty of time."

I knew that the tomatoes and peppers would need to be planted in mid April and that the seedlings would take four to six weeks to mature before setting. Any wait would delay our planting and reduce our yield. I told Pop this and he looked confused. He had forgotten the planting rule that he had repeated to me, over and over, through the years... you plant your garden after the tax man comes. His lapse of memory was just another reminder of the urgency of this garden.

Accepting my explanation he immediately began to tell me where his flower pots were and how we could plant the seeds in those. I let him go through the process before I told him of my plan. I said "Pop, I bought peat starter pots for the seeds this year and potting soil that already contains fertilizer and vermiculite. This will save us time when we set the plants." He thought about this for a minute and I could tell that he didn't want to change the way he had done this for years. Finally he said, "Well, we can plant our seeds in those, but I have promised some plants to L.D. Bell and Bud Forbes at the church. Maybe we can do theirs in the flower pots." A compromise had been reached, but I had this nagging fear that my high tech solution would be proven inferior.

As I filled the peat containers with potting soil, Pop disappeared into the house. He returned shortly with a large mailing envelope full of seeds. I finished the pots while he laid the packets of seeds out on the swing beside him, and called to Grandma for a permanent marker. We were finally going to start our gardening.

I poured the first packet of tomato seeds into the palm of my hand and asked him how deep to plant them. He slowly bent over and poked a finger into the first pot. "Plant them this deep" he said, and I proceeded to poke similar holes in each pot.

As I dropped the first few seeds into their holes, I remarked about how small the seeds were and wondered aloud about the possibility of them germinating. Pop sat patiently listening and then said "ninety percent of them will come up, and you will be surprised how much God can stuff into such a small seed." I stopped what I was doing and looked into his eyes, they were wet with tears, and I quietly thanked God for allowing me to be with this man. He has turned our garden into a lesson on life, one I will cherish forever.

The planting went slowly and all the while, Pop would tell me exactly how many tomatoes and peppers it would take to make a row in the garden. It was a special afternoon with a gardener that grew plants and tutored a son-in-law.

Once all of the peat pots were planted, I placed the trays into the green house and started on the flower pots for L.D. and Bud. I must admit that they were much easier to plant, even if the process wasn't quite as precise as mine. Somehow I knew that these seeds stood a better chance of survival, but I couldn't explain why. I just knew that they were touched by the master gardener.

I watered each pot with warm water, as instructed, before finally announcing that we were done. Pop looked pleased and told me that in about a week we would see young plants poke their heads from the soil. The wrinkles in his face framed a smile that his eyes mirrored. I knew in my heart that this was a day well spent.

Tuesday, March 13, 2007

I had lunch today with Jason Barrett, a good friend, coworker, and bi-vocational Baptist Minister. We stopped by the Young's to see if my seed trays needed watering. Jason had met Pop on several occasions and knew that he was a gardener. Jason is also a gardener, and has been since he was in diapers. His family has always had a garden, and helping his grandfather the previous year with his garden was one of Jason's treasured memories.

We looked at the garden before returning to work, and found that it needed to be tilled again. Over the winter weeds had once again covered the ground. I had also left the weeds in the strawberries until spring. Jason volunteered to help me till and weed the garden during lunch the next day. I was glad for the help and took him up on the offer.

<u>Wednesday, March 14, 2007</u>

Jason and I brought old shoes and clothes to work in anticipation of a lunch outing to the garden. The morning passed slowly, but after an eternity it finally arrived. Jason grabbed his clothes and boots and we headed for the parking lot.

Arriving at Pop's, we found that L.D. Bell and Bud Forbes were there visiting. They had brought Pop the yellow tomato seeds they had promised. These were seeds from plants that Pop had given L.D. the year before. They were special because the original plants had come from Pop's hometown, Sparta Tennessee.

Jason and I changed and went to the garden. Jason would weed the strawberries and I would run the tiller. Typical of early season work, we found that there wasn't gas for the tiller. No problem, a quick trip to the gas station and we were in business. The tiller started right up and purred like a kitten.

I made close passes down the rows of strawberries and Jason began his weeding. We commented on the number of surviving plants, as I moved on to the rest of the garden.

We had only been working a short while when Pop showed up at the garden's edge. He made his way to the folding chair that he had sat dejectedly in during the past season, and watched us as we worked. Occasionally he would use his cane to reach out and break a clod of dirt that had been left by the tiller. The melancholy was gone.

With the garden tilled and weeded we went to the house to change and wash up. Pop was sitting in his swing on the patio. I told him that the garden looked a little better now and he replied "It looks a lot better." As I started to walk for the back door, Pop stopped me. "Rich, can you go up back and bring me a pot for these tomato seeds?"

I retrieved a pot from the back fence line and filled it with potting soil. Knowing he would fall if he bent over, I placed it on a chair for him and told him that I would come back after work to water and put it in the greenhouse. The last thing I wanted was for him to get hurt, especially in his feeble state.

Jason and I returned to work. As we drove, Jason told me that our lunchtime gardening reminded him of working with his grandfather. Quietly, I was hoping that Pop would see the culmination of our efforts. Jason and I were both lost in our thoughts. It was a special day shared by friends.

The Quickening

The term, quickening, refers to the very first signs of life. It is the first movement of a child in the womb, or in the case of a garden, it is the very first sign of life in a seed. With the quickening comes the anticipation of new life in all its glory.

The vision of the once barren garden, growing lush and green, yielding baskets of vegetables, is now with me always. The excitement of the endeavor overshadows the hours of work that will go into the project, and seeing Pop this upbeat again is invigorating.

Saturday, March 17, 2007

I was in an art store with my wife Ann when my cell phone rang, it was Pop and his tone was dire. He began, "Rich we have a problem in the greenhouse!" I immediately had visions of fire, or some accident of epic proportion. Quickly I asked, "what's going on Pop?" to which he responded, "There is too much water in the seed trays and our seeds are going to rot!" After exhaling a deep sigh of relief, I told him that I would be right over. He seemed relieved that I was on the way and that we would handle the crisis.

Ann was looking at me with intense interest as I closed my cell phone. "What's going on?" she asked, and I proceeded to fill her in on the greenhouse problem. Ann gave me a sad smile; she had seen these crises on a number of occasions. She is the caregiver who takes her parents to the doctor and handles all of their health related issues. I dropped her off at our house and went straight way to Pop's.

He met me at the door and followed me to the greenhouse, the tone of urgency still in his voice. When I stepped into the greenhouse, I saw the problem immediately. All of the flower pots that we had planted in Pop's traditional manner were full of small green tomato plants, while those planted in my peat pots were soggy, wet, and showed no life.

I had watered the pots equally, but the deeper flower pots had been able to absorb more water. The peat pots had drained down into the tray they were sitting in and were completely soaked to the point of being muddy. "This is my fault" I told Pop, but he responded that it wasn't anyone's fault, and that if there was any chance of saving the seeds we needed to dry these pots out immediately. I started working quickly.

The black plastic trays contained over an inch of water in them and the peat pots were wicking it up. I sat each pot onto the concrete floor of the greenhouse and emptied the water from the plastic trays. Pop recommended leaving them out of the trays for a while and I agreed.

With the peat pots draining, I asked Pop if he thought the seeds were ruined. He didn't know the answer to this question, but asked me what we would do if they were. I had formulated a plan for that very situation as I drove to Pop's house. I told him that I would go to the local Loews, or Co-Op, and buy replacement seeds. They might not be the exact variety that he had painstakingly selected from the seed catalog, but they would be close. I told him that if we didn't see plants in a couple of days, that we would replant the pots with the new seeds. At worst we would lose a week in our planting. Pop agreed that this was the only solution. I didn't voice my fail safe plan, but if it came down to it, I would buy seedlings and we would use them.

Pop and I walked back into the house and discussed the best places to find seeds locally. I would try to match the varieties as closely as I could. It saddened me to know that I had screwed up at this early stage of our garden. Suddenly I realized that Pop had taught me several unintended lessons. He had taught me that water, although necessary, could be overdone. He taught me the importance of drainage in pots, and he taught me that gardening required adapting to situations as they arise.

As I was saying my goodbyes, I looked at Pop and said, "I hope that you have learned something from this." He looked puzzled and asked "how's that?" I smiled and said that he would need to watch me much closer than he had anticipated. He laughed.

Sunday, March 18, 2007

Pop called me this evening to discuss acquiring new seeds. He had forgotten our conversation from the previous day. I patiently listened as he rehashed our plan, and told him that I would get the seeds. Somewhat saddened, I hung up the phone, but this is why I wanted to plant the garden; Pop's joy, realized through my persistence and patience.

Monday, March 19, 2007

I visited the Lawn and Garden section of our local Loews store today and purchased replacement seeds. I was able to find all but one variety contained in Pop's original order. He was happy to hear that I had found the seeds and immediately remembered the one variety that I had been unable to find. I am always amazed that his once incredible memory can be so keen at times, only to slip away later. I do realize however that when it comes to gardening, his memory is better than usual.

Thursday, March 22, 2007

I made a quick lunchtime visit to the greenhouse today and replanted all of the pots that didn't show signs of life. Jason helped me while Pop gave us instruction.

The flower pot of yellow tomato seeds didn't have a single plant, so Pop asked me to replant it with Early Girl tomatoes. He was very disappointed because of the special meaning that these plants had to him. He dreaded calling L.D. to inform him that none of the yellow seeds had germinated.

Jason and I quickly replanted and I watered the pots carefully before leaving. This time I made certain not to over water.

Friday, March 23, 2007

Pop called and asked me when we had replanted the pots. I told him that it was yesterday, and he informed me that the planter of yellow tomato seeds was full of new plants. I laughed out loud at the irony. Pop's plants must have been just below the surface as I reseeded the planter. I told him that I would either transfer, or pull up the Early Girls when they broke the surface. Pop was adamant that we transfer them to other pots. Killing a plant intentionally was just something he couldn't do.

I hung up the phone with a smile on my face. The good Lord was making certain that I didn't screw up this job. The miracle of life had withstood my clumsy efforts.

Saturday, March 24, 2007

I woke my son Chris at what was an incredibly early 8:30 to begin a day in Pop's garden. This is much later than my 5:30 rising, but for a college student, it is a very early Saturday morning.

We climbed into Chris' truck and headed to the Fairview Co-Op where I purchased four bales of straw, five bags of fertilizer, two bags of lime, some weed killer, and a pound each of Silver Queen corn, Early Contender bush beans, and Roma II bush bean seeds.

We talked about various subjects as we drove to Pop's house to begin our day. The plan was to clean out the gutters, mow the lawn, till the garden a final time, and to straw the strawberry plants. I was glad to have Chris helping me. He is a strapping young man who can work all day without showing much wear at all.

Chris began mowing the yard as I climbed onto the roof and blew the leaves out of the gutters. My job went quickly and in a short time I was cranking the tiller at the garden. No sooner than the tiller began to purr, Pop arrived to take his seat at the fence row. He watched intently as I ran the tiller up and over the pile of composted leaves. They were now a dark soil, rich and black. Pop wants to plant cantaloupes and watermelons here, and let them grow up and over the raised pile. I had made several passes when a tire on the tiller broke its bead. I hadn't noticed that the tire was low before I started.

I pulled the tiller down to the house and Pop told me where he kept his electric air compressor. Chris noticed me working and came to my aid. He wrapped a strap around the tire and tightened it with a wrench. This forced the tire back onto its bead. I attached the compressor to the valve stem, but the air flow wasn't strong enough to overcome the small amount of air that seeped out as it pumped.

We were ready to give up and load the tiller into the truck for a ride to the gas station when Pop's neighbor Jason came over with his compressor. It was much stronger and in a short amount of time the tire was inflated. I thanked Jason, telling him that he had saved us much time. This garden has many friends.

As I tilled, Chris finished the yard and came to my assistance. I told him that Pop would instruct him on what needed to be done to the strawberries. Pop had once again taken his seat at the edge of the garden, and was watching as the job progressed.

Under Pop's tutelage, Chris fertilized, limed, and spread straw on the rows of strawberries. They had already blossomed, so he had to be very careful. He didn't want to knock the blossoms off. In short order, Chris had the two rows of dark green plants looking like they had never lacked for attention.

With the garden ready for planting, we gathered our tools and cleaned up the equipment. Pop was adamant about cleaning every tool before it was stored. We were careful to insure that everything was returned to its place, and at 3:30, we were done for the day.

Monday, March 26, 2007

Pop called this evening to tell me that his son, Don, had stopped by, and that he had watered the seedlings in the greenhouse. I smiled to myself and told him "that's great." I knew that Don had probably stopped by for another reason and had been commandeered for the job of watering. God blesses even the reluctant volunteers.

Tuesday, March 27, 2007

Pop called and asked me if I could pick up another bag of potting soil. He wanted to transplant the yellow tomato seedlings into individual pots. What he said next distressed me greatly.

He went on to tell me that he and Grandma had moved some of the flats around in the greenhouse. Both Grandma and Pop are too unsteady on their feet to be in the greenhouse. It worries me that Pop is trying to engage himself beyond his ability. In order to work in the greenhouse you must stand on a steep set of concrete steps (leading to the basement) and one fainting spell or misstep could mean disaster. I resolved myself to the fact that I would have to discuss this with him, and that he might get his feelings hurt. I know however, that if he or Grandma were to fall, I would have to answer to Ann, her brothers, and my conscience.

I will wait to get the potting soil until I can be there for the repotting. If I pick it up and deliver it to Pop's house, he will be back in the greenhouse and probably have Grandma standing on those stairs as well. The thought of them falling disturbs me greatly.

Thursday, March 29, 2007

Pop called Ann this morning and was very concerned that the temperature in the greenhouse had climbed too high. He was afraid that the seedlings would roast. Ann had plans for the day and I was at work, so my daughter Holly took my one year old granddaughter, Jane Ann, and went to rescue the tomatoes.

Holly and Jane Ann had a wonderful afternoon. They moved the flats of young plants onto the patio and went to the garden to plant a few strawberry sets in gaps where weeds had strangled plants. Jane Ann had the time of her life throwing dirt and helping Mommy.

Later in the afternoon Holly's husband Josh joined them and put potting soil into several dozen pots. Pop wanted to transplant the yellow tomatoes from the large container into individual pots.

Pop called this evening to tell me how wonderful it was to have them helping. He went on and on about Jane Ann throwing dirt and running around in the back yard. Pop and the garden were reaching out to new generations.

Saturday, March 31, 2007

I was up early this morning and after several cups of coffee (late night following my son Jim's Rugby game), I headed over to Pop and Grandma's to plant strawberry sets before rain moved in. A line of storms was due to arrive in the evening and it would make it impossible for me to get into the garden.

I pulled into Pop's driveway and to my amazement; the grass had grown to the point that it needed to be mowed again. I walked in and greeted Grandma. Pop was on the patio sitting in his swing so I walked out the back door and called his name. The response was immediate and cheerful.

I went over my plans for the day with him. First I would mow the yard and then set the strawberries. He was excited about the prospect and told me that we would need a row about three feet from the existing strawberries. I agreed and before I could walk off, he asked me to fetch a quart of fertilizer and lime from the shed so that he could put it on our tomato seedlings before he watered them.

I told Pop that I would bring down the fertilizer and lime, but as I was heading to the shed, he said, "these plants are not growing like I thought they would, they should be bigger after 4 or 5 weeks." This caught me off guard, because I knew when we had planted them. I thought for a moment and said, "Pop, we only planted them a little over two weeks ago." He looked confused and I knew that he had lost track of the days. This is something he would never have done even two years ago. I told him that the fertilizer and lime would do nothing but help, and went on to the shed to get it.

After leaving the pots of fertilizer and lime on the patio, I cranked up the yard tractor and began mowing. It was a gorgeous day and the job went fast. I finished the front yard and while mowing the back yard, I saw Pop bending over the tomato seedlings with a watering can. I felt warm inside as I watched him feebly move from one pot to the next. He was gardening, and we were a team.

I finished the yard and took the strawberry plants to the garden. I had set a couple when I saw Pop leaving the patio with the aid of his walker. He was stooped more than usual and I went to help him as he traversed the back yard. Some days are better than others for him and today wasn't a good one. He labored hard to reach the garden and I held his arm as he walked. He never wants me to help him beyond this.

When we reached the garden, Pop was looking down at the ground. He never made eye contact, but said "Rich, I need to go back to the house. I shouldn't have tried to walk up here; it's a lot further than I thought." I told him that I would help him back to the house and even though he told me that he didn't want to interrupt my planting; I insisted. On the shuffling walk back to the patio, Pop kept apologizing for keeping me from my work. Finally, I looked at him and said, "Pop, I'm here because of you, not these plants. There is plenty of time for them."

We reached the patio and he was obviously exhausted and hurting. To complain isn't in his character, but he told me that his neck hurt. I asked him if the pain felt like soreness, or a crick, and he responded "a crick." I tried to take him into the house, but he insisted that he wanted to sit on his swing where he could see me in the garden.

Pop's Garden Gift

I helped him into the swing and sat down across from him in a lawn chair. Pop said, "I'm OK now, you can go back to your planting" but I insisted that I needed a break and would stay with him for a while. I knew that he wasn't well and wanted to be with him until I was sure that he had recovered from his walk across the yard.

Pop continued to insist that he was fine and that I could go back to my gardening, but I told him that I was thirsty and that I would sit with him and drink something before I planted the rest of the sets. Finally, he seemed alright with this because he felt I was the one who needed the break.

We sat on the patio for a while and talked about how well the original strawberry plants were doing. They were covered in blooms and had sprouted new runners. There would be strawberries galore, and the efforts to reclaim the plants had now born fruit.

After a few minutes, Pop had regained his strength and I went back to the garden. Periodically he would call up to me with a question. "Do you have enough sets for a full row?" or, "those are good looking plants aren't they?" I would yell back from the garden while continuing to plant.

When the final plant had been set, I had a full row of strawberries eighty feet long, and had even planted the additional plants, so as to use all of the sets that had been shipped to us. I gathered and cleaned all of the tools before sitting down across from Pop. He wanted to hear about how the planting went and discuss the coming rain. I enjoyed our conversation and knew this was the best part of the day.

We talked about many things while sitting there on the patio and it will always be a fond memory for me. The view of the garden lined with white blooming dogwoods and Pop passing on bits of wisdom.

The garden I had wanted to plant was now yielding the fruit that I needed most; time with a man I admired.

I left for home at 4:45 in the afternoon, tired, but satisfied with my efforts. The garden was growing more than strawberries; it was nurturing me as well.

Tuesday, April 3, 2007

The weather forecast this morning predicted severe thunderstorms and dropping temperatures. The storms will arrive this evening and then the temperatures will drop back into the fifties with frost warnings at night. This cold snap is anticipated to last for at least the next five days.

Pop called at 9:30 this morning to confirm my thoughts. The seedlings would need to be moved back into the greenhouse. The tender shoots would die if frost were to hit them. I stopped by during my lunch hour and put the trays of plants back into the greenhouse.

Thursday, April 5, 2007

I had just shut off my office computer when the phone rang. It was Pop and he cheerfully informed me "Rich, Our plants are hungry." I laughed and asked if they were getting dry and he said that they were.

I needed to pick up my son Jim from rugby practice after school and told Pop that I would be over later in the evening. He sounded a bit disappointed when he said "that's good." I knew that he wanted me to come over and talk. Watering the plants is always a good excuse for company.

I picked up my son and dropped him off at home before heading to Pop's house. It was 6:00 PM and there was still plenty of light. I wanted to get the seedlings watered while I could still see well.

When I arrived at Pop's, he was sitting in his chair waiting for me. I walked into the house and he immediately started putting on his shoes. Pop loved to stand by the greenhouse and talk to me as I watered. I helped him put on a jacket so that he wouldn't get chilled. He struggled with the zipper until I asked if I could help and zipped it for him.

As I watered, Pop described how he had previously fertilized, limed, and watered the plants. He went on to tell me how they had grown so much since then. Pop had forgotten that I had brought him the containers of fertilizer and lime, and that I had watched him from the garden as he sprinkled the plants with water. I continued to water and pretended that this was the first time I had heard the story. He was proud of his contribution and accomplishment. I was glad to be there.

<u>Friday, April 6, 2007</u>

Ann called me at work this morning to tell me that Pop had phoned to tell her that the small window at the top of the greenhouse needed to be closed. The temperature tonight was going to dip even further into the low twenties and he was afraid the greenhouse might get too cold.

I made my usual trip to the greenhouse, with Jason Barrett, during lunch and closed the window. The greenhouse registered a toasty ninety degrees.

We walked up to the garden for a quick look, and the new strawberry plants I had set were sporting bright new leaves. The original plants were still covered with blooms, but some of the plants now had small green strawberries on them.

Sunday, April 8, 2007

The last two nights have set records as the coldest recorded in Nashville during April. Both nights were in the low twenties and I worry about the strawberries.

Pop called to tell me that his youngest son Joe had mowed the yard and that he did a great job. He told me how much he enjoyed the visit. Joe lives in Atlanta, and with four small children he doesn't have time to visit often. I was glad Joe had spent the time with him.

Pop ended the conversation with "you know our plants could use a drink of water!" to which I laughingly replied, "I'll be there at lunch tomorrow!"

Monday, April 9, 2007

I zipped over to Pop's to water the plants in the greenhouse and grandma met me with a very concerned look on her face.

"Rich, can you check on Alton? He had a bad night and hasn't been able to get out of bed."

I went to the bedroom and Pop was sleeping soundly. Although it was 11:20 in the morning, I didn't want to wake him, so I went back to the kitchen to get the details from Grandma. As she was filling me in on the fact that he was awake much of the night and had been complaining about his stomach being sore, I heard him trying to get up.

I hurried to the bedroom and he was sitting on the side of the bed. I asked him if he wanted to get up and he responded yes. I helped him to his feet and then to the bathroom. His movements were stiff and much slower than normal. I stood by the door as he used the restroom. Pop had heard my voice and didn't want me to see him in bed. His pride wouldn't stand for that.

When he was through in the restroom, I helped him to his recliner and talked with him about his sore stomach. I theorized that transplanting the seedlings several days ago may have caused this. I knew that he couldn't be allowed to do that type of work again. I would have to find creative ways to keep him from joining the work.

Pop shared with me that he didn't think that he could make the doctor's appointment he had with Dr. Van Deveder tomorrow morning. I assured him that we could get him a wheel chair and tried to convince him that this appointment was important. After several minutes he agreed with me, but I felt that he was just trying to placate me and change the subject.

Once I was certain that Pop was alright, and helped him take his medicine, I told him that I would water the plants and come back in to see him. He told me that they really looked great and that the fertilizer and lime he had put on them had helped. I nodded in agreement as I left the room.

I watered the plants and thought about how Pop might never see these plants in the garden. It hurt to entertain such an idea, but the reality was more evident than ever. He was failing by the day. I consoled myself with the fact that he had good days and bad… but today was an exceptionally bad day.

"Lord, let us have him till harvest time. Please give him this garden. Please give me this garden."

Tuesday, April 10, 2007

My cell phone rang while I was on the way to work this morning. Ann's excited voice informed me that Pop had fallen in the shower and Grandma couldn't get him up. My mind raced through my morning appointments and I quickly concluded that regardless of appointments, I needed to immediately go to Pop's house.

A mere 8 minutes later I pulled into the driveway, slammed the car into park and ran into the house. Grandma was calling for help from the bathroom. As I turned from the hallway into the bathroom I could see her predicament. She was holding Pop upright on the closed toilet seat and he was leaning precariously against her.

Moving quickly, I relieved Grandma and balanced Pop's naked body. I asked him how he felt and if he was hurt. His response was weak, but reassuring. "No I'm not hurt, but I can't get up." He went on to say that he needed to lay down.

Holding him securely under each arm I lifted him to his feet. He was able to shuffle his feet very slowly with the added support I was giving. We made it to his bedroom and I lifted him onto the bed. "Just let me lay here a minute" he said as I asked Grandma for a set of underclothes. Pop looked weak and pale, and he was bleeding from a small scrape on his knee. Working quickly, but gently, I dressed him and placed a Band-Aid on his scrape. If an ambulance were to become necessary, I didn't want him to feel embarrassed.

He seemed to be recovering from the episode as I continued to hold his hand and talk to him. It became evident that a 9-1-1 call wouldn't be necessary. Besides, he had a doctor's appointment already scheduled for this morning.

Pop insisted that he didn't think he could make it to his appointment, but I convinced him that between Ann and me, we could get him there. I further told him that the doctor needed to see him now, rather than later. He eventually agreed.

Once Pop was dressed for the doctor and resting comfortably atop the bed, I took a seat beside him and continued to comfort and talk to him. I could tell that he was recovering quickly because his conversation shifted. Out of the blue he looked at me and said, "I saw on the news that several people had lost their tomato plants during the cold snap. I can't believe they set them out this early." Recognizing his need to redirect attention from the earlier fall to something more uplifting, I replied that they obviously didn't understand Nashville weather very well. The garden continued to be Pop's refuge; even when his world was falling down around him.

The doctor visit with Ann went relatively well. Doctor Van Devender adjusted his medication and found that the pain in his stomach was due to shingles. I must admit that I was relieved to hear that our gardening hadn't contributed to his health problems. I must plant our seedlings at the earliest moment possible. I fear that time is short.

<u>Monday, April 16, 2007</u>

Pop called me at the office today to tell me how much the tomato seedlings had grown. He said that he had wanted to sit outside the greenhouse and watch them, but that it was just too chilly for him. I am always amazed at how much he loves plants and gardening.

I remembered last summer as I watched him sit in the garden and stare at the weed infested and withering plants. The fresh new growth in the greenhouse must be invigorating for him. I can't wait to begin planting.

Planting Time

Planting the garden is a much anticipated event to a gardener. All of the plants that have been so caringly grown in greenhouses and cold frames are set into the ground with hopes of bountiful harvest. This is a time of promise; A time of dreams, excitement, and high expectation.

<u>Thursday, April 19, 2007</u>

I was sitting in front of the television set when the phone rang. I looked at the caller ID and saw that it was Pop, and answered immediately. When Pop calls it can be an emergency or just a casual gardening conversation; you never know.

This call was regarding the garden. He reminded me that the tomato seedlings needed to be moved outside, and that his yard needed mowing. Jokingly he added "we've got to adjust your salary," and laughed. I laughed too and said "I think you pretty much have my salary where you want it," at which we both laughed heartily. Pop knew that I wouldn't take any money for helping him, but he brought the subject up often and I knew that he would rather be doing these jobs himself.

Our conversation slipped to tomatoes, and Pop asked me if I knew where Brandywine Tomatoes were developed. I told him no and his voice took on an air of excitement as he went on. "They were developed by the Amish over forty years ago. They can grow to over a pound each and have stood the test of time. I read this in my garden catalog." I was amazed and told him so. He sounded pleased that he could tell me something that I hadn't known before.

I confirmed that I would be over at lunch tomorrow to move the plants outside, and that on Saturday I would mow his grass and plant the corn and bean seeds in the garden. He said "OK Rich see you then" and our call ended. Sitting there in my chair, I felt glad that Planting time was actually here after months of preparation.

Friday, April 20, 2007

Pop and Grandma weren't home when I arrived to move the tomatoes out of the greenhouse. Jason Barrett and I went around back and as I handed the flats of seedlings out of the greenhouse, Jason laid them on the patio. The job was proceeding smoothly until I picked up one flat and noticed that several of the plants had white aphids on them. The plants didn't look as robust as the others and this had drawn my attention.

I showed the aphids to Jason and told him that I would need to pick up some spray before I came out to do yard work tomorrow. Jason agreed that this would be a good idea.

Once back at the office I browsed the web and found that Bonide Rotenone Insect Control, and Shultz Garden Insect Spray were recommended as good applications for aphids.

I'll call Pop tonight and talk to him about this to see what wisdom he can share.

Saturday, April 21, 2007

My biological alarm sounded early this morning, and I immediately dressed and started a pot of coffee. Today I will plant the first seeds of the season in the garden, and although I don't want to arrive at Pop's before 10:00, the anticipation is killing me. In their younger years, my in-laws were early risers, but now they move much slower in the mornings.

I knew that the yard needed mowing before I could begin in the garden, and as I drank my final cup of coffee; I decided to wake my youngest son Jim to help with the yard work. To my amazement, he jumped right out of bed and seemed anxious to help. Stranger things have happened, but I just can't remember when… I waited patiently as he dressed and ate a bowl of cereal. A short drive later we pulled into Pop's driveway, and went inside. Pop was sitting in his recliner and was pleasantly surprised to see Jim with me.

I told him that my plan was to mow the yard and then till enough of the garden to plant three rows of Silver Queen corn and two rows of bush beans. He thought about this a moment and said that we needed to re-pot some of the tomato seedlings. The seeds I had planted in those new fangled peat pots were cramped and not growing like they should. I was a bit disappointed that my work in the garden would be delayed, but after all, the master of the garden knew best. I said "OK" as Jim and I headed for the mowers.

I put Jim on the John Deere riding mower and took the trim mower for myself. I thought that I could clean up any spots that Jim missed as I trimmed around the beds and trees. As it turned out, Jim did a great job and I didn't have to do any additional trimming. We worked quickly and by noon the yard looked great. Our only deviation was to skip the area in front of the bee hives. My brother-in-law, David Young, had replaced two of the hives with new bees and they were very aggressive.

With the yard work finished, Jim and I went to the patio to survey the seedlings and determine what needed to be replanted. Pop was already there sitting on his swing and gave us our marching orders. All of the plants in the smaller (eight cup planters) would need to be transplanted. This amounted to five trays of tomatoes or a total of 160 plants.

Sizing up the job, I developed a plan. Jim would fill one quart pots with potting soil and have them ready for me as I transplanted. We worked steadily for over two hours repotting the plants. It was immediately obvious what the problem was; the little plants were root bound. My carefully selected peat pots had been too small. Another lesson painfully learned. I should have listened to Pop's advice when we planted the seeds.

Grandma came out of the house several times as we worked and offered us lunch, but I insisted on working on. The garden was calling and my time was limited. At one point I looked around and Jim had disappeared; He had slipped into the house for a sandwich. Finally, all of the seedlings were happily in their new containers, and it was time to move to the garden. I was ready to begin gardening in earnest.

I walked along the edge of the garden to pull the roto-tiller from the shed and was immediately attacked by the new aggressive bees. I ran and swatted until clear of the garden. I knew that the problem would be even worse once I started the tiller. The throbbing of the engine would excite the bees into a frenzy.

I went back to the house where Pop was sitting with Jim. He had seen what happened and asked me what I was going to do. Not knowing how to handle this, I suddenly recalled that David had left a bee suit in the tool room. It would be incredibly hot, but would keep me from being stung.

Once suited up in the bee suit and hood, I once again went to the garden. Bees immediately darted around my head. I pulled the tiller out of the shed and started it easily. Just as I thought, the bees were incensed and their activity increased.

I turned the tiller towards my first row and noticed that Pop and Jim had taken seats at the far side of the garden. Instinctively I knew that the bees would follow me across the garden and instructed Jim to get Pop out of there if the bees started coming at them. I was very concerned that Pop wouldn't be able to move away from them in his diminished state and encumbered by his walker.

The first pass across the garden went smoothly and the bees seemed to stay with the tiller. They were particularly attracted to the black handles. As I made my turn near Pop and Jim, I kept my eye on them. Any sign of attack and I would leave the tiller and help Jim get Pop out of there. As it turned out, Jim killed a couple of bees, but the bulk of the little defenders stayed with me and the throbbing tiller. I worked about twenty five feet of the garden into a smooth texture before returning the tiller to the shed. I was sweating profusely in the stifling bee suit and needed a break.

Before leaving the garden, I went to the rows of strawberries where I had notice a gleam of red below the dark green leaves as I was tilling. Sure enough, there was a plump red strawberry; the first of the season. I picked it and walked over to Pop. When I extended my hand, and he saw the berry, his eyes lit up. He gently took it from me and critiqued the berry. "That's a good looking berry isn't it?" He said while tuning it in his hand. Then he slowly brought it to his mouth and bit off the stem. He paused a moment before placing the berry into his mouth. The look on his face was priceless. Then, as if he were tasting a strawberry for the first time, "That's so sweet" he said to himself. God had allowed him to taste the bounty of his garden again.

As I walked back to the house the bees returned to the hive. I couldn't believe how aggressive they had been. Pop and Jim had retreated to the patio by the time I joined them there. I quickly shed the hot suit and felt the cool air on my soaked clothing. Jim brought me a cold drink as I sat with Pop on the patio. I needed to replenish the fluid I had lost.

It was six o'clock and there wasn't time to put any seeds in the ground. To tell the truth, I didn't relish the idea of planting while garbed in a bee suit. Pop was concerned about the bees and proposed asking David to move the new hives out to his farm. They were far more aggressive than the existing hives had been.

We sat in the cool evening breeze and discussed what needed to be done next. I told Pop that I would come back tomorrow and plant our seeds. This might give the bees a chance to calm down. Our day was done and I felt like we had accomplished much; father, son-in-law, and grandson.

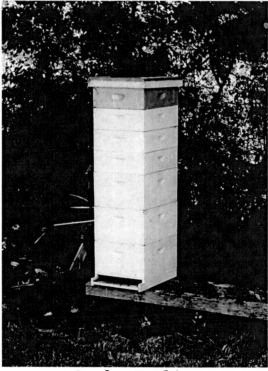
Garden Beehive

Sunday, April 22, 2007

It was early morning when I arrived at Pop's house. I wanted to get started planting the garden while it was still cool. Hopefully the bees would be more lethargic, and I wouldn't have to don the hot bee suit again.

I retrieved several stakes that I would use to mark my rows, and after careful measurements, I ran string down my rows. Three feet between every row, five rows in all. I took a hoe and created a narrow trench using the string to keep them straight. I knew that Pop wouldn't like a wavy row.

The bees made frequent visits, but I found that if I held my breath and didn't raise my head, that they would buzz around then leave. The moment I exhaled they would be back. It was a touchy game we played. I received several stings, but they didn't penetrate my clothing. The bees would sting and then drop in the soil to die.

After the trenches were created, I planted my seeds. First were the rows of Silver Queen corn. I planted eight seeds per foot of row; three rows in all. Next I planted the two rows of beans. Each row of beans was divided, a half row of Roma II, and a half row of Early Contender. These seeds were planted every two inches. Once the seeds have sprouted, I will thin them. The corn will be thinned to one plant per foot, while the beans will be thinned to no more than one plant every six inches.

As I was planting the beans, I decided to plant each row by planting half the row in one type bean and then finishing the row with the other. At harvest time I will be able to sit on a bucket between the two rows and pick a certain variety of beans without as much effort. To find the center of the row, I had to pace off the distance and then divide that number of paces by two. As I paced off my row to place a stake in the center, I happened to look up… On the edge of the garden stood a small dogwood tree; it was precisely in the center of the garden. Pacing wasn't necessary. Pop had planted it to use as a landmark. This was a trick he had learned as a child on the farm.

After all of the seeds were in their rows and covered with soil, I joined Pop on the patio. He hadn't attempted to make the trip to the garden today. I think that the previous day's events had sapped his strength. Grandma came out of the house and sat close by his side.

We talked about grandchildren, great grandchildren, and the garden. I said "well the seeds are in the ground, now it's up to God." Pop quickly responded "He'll do his part, he always does." I smiled and was glad to be here with them. They always make sense of life and show me what is truly important.

Monday, April 23, 2007

Pop called me this afternoon and wanted me to stop by his house on the way home from work. Apparently he had visitors today and they all want some tomato plants. Pop felt that we should set aside the plants we need for our garden. I did some quick math and we will need eighty one plants for our three rows, plus some spares in case we lose plants. All in all, I figure one hundred plants will be more than enough for us.

I want to bring a few plants to Jason Barrett since he has helped me plant, water, and care for the seedlings over the past several weeks. Those who participate get preferential treatment.

I arrived at Pop's and found him sitting on the patio behind the house talking with a neighbor as her young sons played merrily around them. After greeting them, I began separating the seedlings into OURS and THEIRS sections. Pop kept pointing to nice plants with his cane and instructing me to "take that big one right there! No not that one... that one! That's right!" After much deliberation, we had selected over one hundred plants for the garden. Eighty one to be planted and the remainder for spares in case we lost a plant to cut worms or disease.

After the plants were divided, I picked out nine healthy seedlings for Jason. He was particularly interested in trying the Brandywine, so I found four nice ones for him. Pop had already slid a flat of eighteen yellow tomatoes to the side for L.D. Bell and Bud Forbes.

I think that Pop's custom of giving plants to friends is a big part of the tradition surrounding his garden. I tasted a bit of the satisfaction that he has savored for all these years when I placed my tray of tomato plants in the bed of Jason Barrett's truck. It is a feeling of being helpful and kind. What a wonderful hobby this is. It reinforces the best of human virtues.

Thursday, April 26, 2007

We had a nice rain last night. I was lying in bed listening as it pattered on the roof when I suddenly realized that I was thinking about the effect of the warm raindrops on our garden. Usually, I was more concerned with whether an umbrella would be needed in the morning.

I silently said a quick prayer of thanks for the rain. Pop had been right, God was doing his part.

Saturday, April 28, 2007

After a day of family activities, I was finally able to sit in my easy chair and relax. I had taken my son Chris to the eye doctor for new glasses and attended the 80th birthday party for Bill Hughes (Pop's brother-in-law).

Not long after I sat down, the phone rang. I picked it up to hear Pop's voice in the receiver. "Rich, we need to get these plants in the ground. What are your plans?" I told him that I would be over in the morning and that Jim and I would mow the yard and set out the tomato plants. Pop was relieved to hear this news. He would often forget our agreements regarding which day I would do something. This was just another case in point.

There was good news during the conversation. David had removed the two new bee hives from Pop's yard. I was glad to hear that a bee suit wouldn't be necessary. Also, Don had been by this morning and dug three bushes out of the upper garden. This would give us more room for the cantaloupes and watermelons.

After hearing that I planned to set out the tomatoes, Pop went on to tell me about a bad fall he had taken. His ribs were bruised from his sternum around to his back. I asked him how this had happened and he informed me that he had fallen while bringing in the groceries. This confused me because I knew the he couldn't lift the bags. He went on to describe how Grandma had set them outside the door and he had taken the crook of his cane and tried to drag the bags into the house. Walking backwards, he had fallen onto a chair.

Sunday, April 29, 2007

Jim and I arrived at Pop's house around 10:00 A.M. and went inside. Pop looked very weak as he sat in his favorite chair. We went over my plans for the day and Pop told me that he wouldn't be able to come outside today. Although there had been times that he hadn't come to the garden, this was the first time he had verbalized his limitation. The fall, coupled with his degenerating health, had exhausted him.

Jim began mowing the yard and I went to the garden to prepare for planting. Two bags of fertilizer were spread over the unplanted portion of the garden and would be worked into the soil. I tilled enough area for three rows of tomatoes. The rows would be 42 inches apart and we would set the plants 36 inches from each other in the rows. My plan was to till the remainder of the garden, but once again a tire broke its bead. Although dissatisfied with not being able to finish tilling, I decided to make the best of the situation. Taking stakes and a tape measure, I drove stakes marking the three rows and strung twine between them to mark my lines.

Jim joined me in the garden for the planting. After a quick lesson on how to plant a tomato seedling, we started. Jim planted one row and I the next. By working this way, I could watch him as he worked beside me. He did a wonderful job and I was proud of my fifteen year old son. The task was much easier with two of us planting together. Having planted all three rows, we stood at the side of the garden and surveyed our work. The lines of plants were straight and uniformly spaced.

With the plants in the ground, we ran a garden hose to the garden and gave the little seedlings their first drink of water in their new home. Jim walked behind me as I watered and kept the hose from knocking over the delicate plants. We were proud of our day's work together.

Monday, April 30, 2007

During my lunch hour, I went to the garden. I was hoping that the plants would be fine, but the day was an exceptionally hot eighty five degrees and the tender leaves were showing signs of wilt. I discussed this with Pop and he reassured me that they would perk up again when the sun went down. He went on to suggest another watering this evening.

Watering in the evening fit perfectly with my plans. My son-in-law, Josh Girdler, was going to bring an air compressor over this evening and help me re-inflate the tiller tire. I decided to arrive a little earlier and water the plants before he arrived.

As for the unplanted seedlings, L.D. Bell and Bud Forbes had visited earlier in the day and taken all of the plants that Pop and I hadn't designated as replacements for our garden. I was glad they had done this because Pop worried about them and tried to tend to them. In his weak state, this was an accident waiting to happen.

L.D. and Bud had also walked Pop to the garden where he saw the young tomatoes standing proudly, as they had for so many years previous. Pop took great pride in telling me how nice the two of them thought the garden looked. No weeds, straight rows, and perfectly spaced plants.

This evening, I went to Loews and picked up a new throttle cable for the tiller. The old one had touched the muffler and melted. This kept the tiller from running at full throttle without my pulling the cable with my hand as I tilled.

Josh met me at Pop's about 7:00 P.M. to fix the deflated tire and helped me install the new throttle cable. We were joined by my wife Ann, daughter Holly, and granddaughter Jane Ann. As we worked on the tiller, I remembered times when Ann and I would watch Pop at the garden. Now there were four generations brought together by this same garden.

Our garden was taking shape, and Pop was proud of it once again. My hours of work and planning were having the effect that I had hoped. Pop was seeing the garden as he had when his own hands held the soil lovingly in them.

Tuesday, May 1, 2007

It's May Day, but there will be no rest for me. I noticed that rain is predicted for the next four days straight. I still need to plant my peppers and the hills of cantaloupes and watermelons.

I worked at the office through the morning, and decided that the coming rain would put me over a week behind in my planting if I didn't do something drastic. I decided to take the afternoon off and head to the garden. With this extra time I plan to till the remaining ground, and plant it.

After changing clothes, I went over my plan to till the remainder of the garden with Pop. He was excited that the end of planting was near and insisted on joining me at the garden to show me where he wanted the cantaloupe and watermelon hills. I convinced him to stay in the house and that I would come get him when I was ready to make the hills. I am afraid to have him out very long because the temperate today is over ninety degrees.

When I finally shut off the tiller, I looked out across the garden. It looked wonderful, even through sweat covered glasses. Not wanting to get Pop quite yet, I decided to stake out a row for the pepper plants. They were small and I would set them out later in the evening to avoid the heat of the day.

Finally I had done all that I could do without Pop showing me where he wanted the melon hills. I went to the house and he asked me to help him put on his shoes and find his walker. In short order we were traversing the back yard.

I wanted to take Pop up the shady side of the yard, but he insisted on being closer to where I would be working. We walked slowly past the beehive and I sat him beside the garden on a folding chair. From this vantage point, Pop directed me to where he wanted the hills made and instructed me on precisely how to make and plant them.

Upon completion of the melon hills, I helped Pop to his feet and we started back towards the house. It didn't take long before I realized that he was struggling. The heat had taken its toll and he was barely able to shuffle. As we reached the beehive, Pop's legs gave out on him. We were directly in front of the hive and in the flyway of the bees.

In less than a minute the first guard bee started buzzing us. I knew that we were in a bad position and tried to help Pop back to his feet. He was exhausted and couldn't move. More bees started buzzing around us and in short order they went into attack mode and started stinging us. Knowing that we couldn't stay here without becoming covered in bees, I took drastic action. Squatting behind Pop, I placed both of my arms beneath his arm pits and lifted him off the ground. I ran him to safety, apologizing as I went. I kept repeating, "Pop, I hope I'm not hurting you, but we have to get out of here!"

Once clear of the bee's flyway the attack ceased and I was able to set Pop on the ground. He was thanking me profusely, and I was asking him if he was hurt. We both knew that we had barely avoided a potentially dangerous situation. When bees sting they release a pheromone which alerts others in the hive that an attack is occurring and they join the fight to protect the hive. Fortunately, the damage had been minor; two stings each.

After a rest in the shade, I helped Pop back to the house and into his comfortable chair. We talked about the bees and how there couldn't have been a worse place to have stopped. Neither of us blamed the bees for the situation, they were behaving as they would to repel any intruder.

It was nearly four o'clock and I had to pick up my son Jim from rugby practice. I let Pop know that I would be back around six to plant the pepper plants. He said "that's great, I want to take a nap," and I headed off to Franklin High School.

At six o'clock, I pulled back into Pop and Grandma's driveway. The sun was lower and the heat had subsided. I stuck my head in the door to let them know that I was back before proceeding on to the garden. Pop said that he was feeling much better and I felt a rush of relief. I planted the pepper plants, weeded the strawberry plants, and gathered my tools. It was now seven thirty in the evening and I had accomplished all that I had set out to do.

Inside the house, I could smell the cornbread that Grandma had baked for dinner. She is a tremendous cook and her meals are prepared in high Southern fashion. Pop and Grandma were sitting in the family room when I joined them. Pop smiled and asked me "Is the garden layed by?" Looking at him quizzically, I asked "What?" he said again, "Is the garden layed by?" Seeing the look on my face he offered an explanation, "when I was growing up in the country, a farmer would say that he had layed a field by when he had plowed it for the last time and planted it." I smiled and said, "Yes sir, the garden is layed by."

We talked together for a brief while. Pop was especially glad that the cantaloupes and watermelons had been planted before the rain arrived. I could tell that these would be his favorites, and made a mental note to myself that they would get special attention.

Pop's Garden Gift

Growing In the Sun While Clouds Gather

Once the garden has been planned, prepared, and planted, there is a time of let down. The weeds haven't begun to grow, the harvest is a ways off, and the vegetable plants are springing out of the ground. One finds themselves waiting for something to do and anticipating the first of the garden's bounty to arrive.

I am amazed at nature's vitality as the plants strengthen and grow. This is a time of rain, sun, and warmth.

Monday, May 7, 2007

After attending a doctor's appointment with my son Jim, who had broken his leg just above the ankle practicing rugby, I decided to call Pop. I need advice on when to thin the beans and corn to the recommended number of plants per row foot. I knew that I could do this job after work today, but with my son having surgery on his leg in the morning, it would be a couple of days if I waited.

Pop answered his phone almost immediately and seemed to be in good spirits. It had rained for the past three days, so I asked him if he thought the garden was dry enough for me to get into it. "No, you will do more damage than good right now, I would wait a couple of days" was his reply. I went on to explain that I needed to thin the beans and corn, but he felt that there was no rush to do this. His recommendation was to wait until the plants were about eight inches tall.

After I hung up, the need to see the garden overcame me. I decided to swing by Pop's on the way home just to look at the garden and to check on Pop and Grandma. It had been a few days since I had dropped in, and I was missing them; Pop, Grandma, and our garden.

After a long day at the office, I stopped by to see them. Grandma and Pop were sitting in their family room when I walked in, and they greeted me immediately.

We had been chatting a few minutes when Pop asked me if I had been up to see the garden. I responded "No," but told him I was heading up that way. He asked me to check on how wet the soil was and if the melons had come up yet.

As I walked to the edge of the garden, I was amazed at how tall the plants had become. It seems that even a couple of days can make such a difference in them. My corn was now about eight to ten inches high, but I noticed that about ten feet of one row was missing. Upon closer inspection it became apparent that a bird had pulled the young plants from the ground and eaten the kernels of corn from under them. I walked to the back of the garden and sure enough, the melon hills were sporting new growth. Tiny young melon plants had reared their heads from the soil.

The moment I entered the house, I called to Pop that the melons were up. He yelled back from the family room "GREAT!" I filled him in on how tall each of our plantings were and gave him the bad news about the birds in the corn. He immediately recommended a scarecrow. While constructing one in my mind, I told him that I would be over this weekend to replant the lost corn, thin the plants, and erect a scarecrow. He thought that was a great idea. I left for home thinking of the best design for a scarecrow. Something I had only seen in books.

Wednesday, May 9, 2007

Ann and I brought Jim home from the hospital today following surgery on his broken ankle. There were multiple messages waiting on the answering machine and Pop and Grandma had left two of them. They were worried about Jim and wanted an update. Ann called to reassure them that he was fine but before hanging up, Pop wanted to speak to me.

When I said hello, Pop began to tell me that his son Don had helped him to the garden today. Much like our last trip, Don and his son Chase had to carry Pop back to the house after his legs lost their strength. The discussion of this episode was only casually mentioned before he started talking about our garden.

Pop had made several observations while at the garden. The strawberries were covered in blooms and berries, the birds had damaged more corn plants, the melons needed to be thinned to two or three plants per hill, the beans and corn could now be thinned, and he reinforced his previous recommendation that a scarecrow was needed as soon as possible! With pride in his voice, he went on to tell me about walking between the tomato rows from one side of the garden to the other. These were the first steps he had made into the garden proper since it was planted. He was at home there and had reestablished his link with this old friend.

Sunday, May 13, 2007

I wasn't able to work the garden this weekend due to my involvement in the Tennessee State High School Rugby Tournament. My cell phone rang while at the pitch and it was Ann. Pop had taken a dramatic turn for the worse. He couldn't remember any of his family, and didn't know that the home he had built and lived in for 54 years was his. The family gathered at the Emergency Room.

While standing at Pop's bedside in the ER, I told him that I was going to be working on the garden this week. He immediately recounted all of the tasks that needed to be done, and reminded me to bring him a pellet rifle so that he could shoot the blackbirds that were raiding the corn. I was amazed that he could remember this so clearly, given that the rest of his life's memories were in shambles. I left the room and Ann asked him about the garden... he couldn't remember a garden.

As I was driving home late in the night, I thought to myself that whatever the outcome, this would be a garden I would forever cherish.

Monday, May 14, 2007

Dr. Karl Van Devender escorted Ann and me to Pop's room in the Intensive Care Unit. He then informed us that Pop had Acute Delirium, but he felt that over time the condition would improve. He was uncertain what had triggered this, but Ann's research indicated that this was a common symptom of advanced congestive heart failure.

Wednesday, May 16, 2007

With Pop in the hospital and Grandma at home alone, I decided to swing by and check on her. When I arrived she was getting dressing to go to the hospital. Susanne Young, David's wife, was coming by to pick her up. I excused myself and headed up to see the garden.

It had been a while since I saw the garden. Most of my time over the past few days had been spent at Centennial Medical Center with Pop or my son Jim. I was pleasantly surprised to see that the garden hadn't missed me too badly. All of the plants had grown considerably, but I did notice that one of the tomato plants looked as if it were struggling. There were few weeds, but

I could tell that there was a slight green tinge between the rows where unwanted plants were trying to establish themselves.

I made mental notes as to what needed to be done this weekend. I would need to till between the rows and hoe around the plants. The corn and beans needed to be thinned out. Stakes need to be driven for the tomato plants and they needed to be tied for the first time. Weed killer needed to be sprayed behind the leaf pile to hold down the growth taking place there, and if I had time, I wanted to plant some hills of yellow squash.

Satisfied that all was well, armed with a to-do list, and reassured that Grandma was fine, I headed back to the office.

Thursday, May 17, 2007

Pop is recovering slowly. Some of his memory has returned, but he is unable to walk or care for himself. I used my lunch hour to visit him.

I walked into Pop's hospital room and thought he was asleep. As I approached the bed, I could tell that his eyes were open and he was looking out the window. It took him a moment to realize that I was there. He turned his face to me and asked where he was. I immediately thought that he had slipped backwards in his recovery, but he continued, "What road is that out there?" I responded "It's Charlotte, Pop." He was satisfied with the answer and began to tell me about his night.

During my visit we discussed the time I thought it would take him to recover, Grandma, the family, and of course the garden.

Later in the evening I was at home tending to Jim. He had caught a stomach virus on top of his broken leg. Ann walked into the house with my son Chris; they had been at the hospital visiting Pop. Apparently the decision had been made to put Pop into a recovery home for rehabilitation. Even though I understood that Grandma couldn't care for him and the necessity of professional help, my heart fell. None of us wanted to see this happen.

Saturday, May 19, 2007

It is Saturday, and while Ann and her brothers are inside Pop's house discussing how best to handle his treatment options; I am working in the garden. He will be moved to a rehabilitation facility to try and strengthen his legs and reestablish his ability to independently provide for his own basic needs. The outcome is uncertain, and Grandma's fragile health will not allow her to tend to him unless he can walk and care for himself.

I lose myself in the garden because this is where I feel closest to Pop. From time to time I look up from my work expecting to see him watching me from the patio. It hurts to see his empty swing. I wonder if I can finish this garden without him, but know that I can't give up on it any more than I can give up on Pop.

I worked on the tasks that Pop and I had discussed. I started by weeding the strawberries. As I worked along, I was joined by Benjamin Young. Benjamin is the 14 year old son of Pop's youngest son Joe. He asked me if he could help, and I put him to work pulling weeds. He was great company and we talked about school, sports, and the life of a 14 year old boy. The garden was reaching out once again to bring family together.

Once the strawberries had been weeded, I pulled the tiller from its shed and began working the garden. I tilled between the rows to remove any small weeds that had started there. The job was slow, but would save a great deal of hand weeding. Once the garden had been tilled I stood back and admired the beauty of the green plants against the dark freshly turned soil. It looked so beautiful that I didn't want to step into it for fear of ruining the image.

I took the four pronged hoe and moved down each row. Being careful not to disturb or damage the young plants, I was able to uproot the small weeds that were starting to grow between them. Pop had told me that this hoe was his favorite tool for the job and it worked perfectly. Not only did it dislodge the weeds, but it broke the crust formed by our last rain. Rain water would easily find its way to the waiting roots.

My next task was to thin the corn plants. There should be one foot between each plant. I remembered Pop telling me to select the healthiest plants and not be overly particular about the spacing. I also needed to transplant several of them to the row that had been damaged by the birds and did so with little effort, lifting them gently with a spade and moving them to a new home.

Although the day was cool, I found myself sweating as I moved along on my knees determining which plants to pull from the ground, which to move to the damaged row, and which to leave standing. The job took quite a while, and I was glad for the mindlessness of it. There is something special about jobs that allow you to wander mentally. By the time I had thinned the corn, it was time to call it a day. I had been working since nine o'clock and it was now four thirty in the afternoon.

As I cleaned my tools and returned them to their proper storage, I thought about what needed to be done tomorrow. I decided that I would thin the beans in the cool of the morning, spray the garden for aphids, and then stake and tie the tomatoes.

Before leaving, I took some pictures of the garden. I want to print them and take them to Pop. I hope that he will enjoy seeing the fruit of our labor, but more than that, I also hope that he will remember what we have done together.

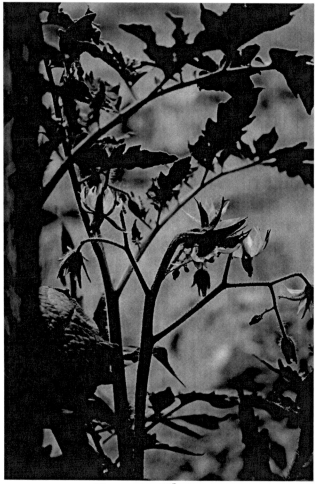
Tomato Blooms

Sunday, May 20, 2007

As anticipated the morning was cool and refreshing. I told Grandma that I would be in the garden most of the day and that if she needed anything to give me a shout. She was glad to have someone there and told me that she was going to my daughter Mariah's baby shower that afternoon. I told her that I would still be there when she returned

I walked up to the garden and started my day by thinning the beans to one plant every six inches. As it turned out, this was a bit harder than working with corn because the stems of the beans were smaller and the leaves hung all the way to the ground. On all fours, I made my way down each row and pulled so many plants that I started feeling wasteful. Once I finished pulling plants, I gathered up the already wilting discards and threw them on the leaf pile to become compost.

After resting for a few moments in Pop's garden chair, I retrieved the Aphid spray from the tool room. The container contained about a gallon of spray and came complete with a hose and spray gun. I read the instructions quickly and walked to the first row of tomatoes. When I squeezed the trigger of what I thought was a pump, a whirring noise was emitted; it was battery operated. I was more than pleased because this would save me from repeatedly squeezing the trigger, like a water pistol, and possibly preclude a sore hand in the morning.

The spraying job went very quickly with my new fangled sprayer and I was able to coat all of the tomato plants, beans, and peppers before I ran out of chemical.

With the spraying completed, I drove to David Young, my brother-in-law's house and borrowed his post driver. This is a tool that slides down over a post and has a handle on each side. You slide the tool up the stake and then let it fall. This drives the stake into the ground without having to swing a hammer, and saves time as well as knuckles.

I returned to Pop's and cut all of his spare stakes to a length of six and one half feet long with a chainsaw before beginning the job of driving them into the dirt beside each plant. The job went smoothly, except for a couple of broken stakes, and before long I had staked forty plants. We had planted more tomatoes than the previous years, and even with the spare stakes that I had cut, there just weren't enough to complete the job.

Once again I was on the phone with David Young and asked him if he could pick up thirty one additional stakes at the saw mill near where he worked. David agreed and after a quick "Thank You," I hung up the phone. Satisfied that there wasn't an alternative solution, I began tying each plant to the stake beside it. Pop had shown me how to tie the plants by passing the string around the stalk then criss-crossing the ends to form a figure eight before tying the other end behind the pole.

After all of the plants were secured to their poles, I sat back down in Pop's garden chair and looked out over the garden. It was beautiful. I was feeling the same satisfaction that Pop had felt for all those years. Pop and I were bound together in a way I found hard to describe. This bond was something basic in ones nature; it was a link to the earth from which God molded Adam.

Monday, May 21, 2007

I walked into the hospital with the pictures that I had taken of the garden. I was wondering how Pop would react to them.

I opened the door to Pop's room and the Physical Therapist was just finishing her session with him. I was amazed to see him standing beside his bed. He was unsteady, but standing none the less. As I moved into the room he sat back into a chair and let out a loud "Whew!" Pop immediately began to tell me about walking out into the hallway and back. The nurse quickly added that he did this with some assistance. Regardless, I could have jumped and clicked my heels!

I handed Pop the pictures of the garden and he was immediately infatuated with them. "The garden looks great" he said while smiling and flipping the pages. He stared intently at each picture and was very excited to hear that I was leaving them for him.

Two different nurses came into the room, and upon seeing the pictures, asked Pop if this was his garden. He would say that it was, and then add, "No it's Rich's garden." I would always tell them that we were a team. He was the brains and I was the brawn. Pop would laugh and tell them that he had worked that garden for many, many, years. He would then describe the plants, and in the case of the tomatoes, he would always add, "there are seventy one."

The orderly brought Pop his lunch and while he ate we made conversation. I told him that the empty area in the back of the garden had been bothering me. His face lit up as he told me that there was a packet of squash seed on his desk at home. I asked him how I should plant them and he told me to make several hills about eighteen inches across and plant three seeds per hill.

I returned after work and, as Pop finished his dinner; we watched the evening weather report. There would be no rain for several days and I was mulling over a plan for watering the garden. Before I could verbalize my concern, Pop said "you will need to water the garden tomorrow; those plants have to be thirsty by now." I smiled to myself because my gardening mentor was instructing me once again. I had missed his guidance so much and had been terrified that I might lose him before his garden bore fruit.

Tuesday, May 22, 2007

Ann called me at the office this afternoon to inform me that Pop was being transferred to a rehabilitation facility as we spoke. He was confused and couldn't understand what was happening and why he couldn't go home. He told Polly Hardwick, his case worker, that he just wanted to walk in his back yard and across the church grounds again. This was his dream; he wasn't acknowledging the fact that he couldn't walk on his own

While watering the garden in the cool of the evening, I thought long about Pop and wondered to myself if there would be a way that I could request a furlough for him. I would like to put him in a wheel chair and push him around the church grounds, and then bring him home to see his yard and garden again. My reservation was that he might become overly melancholy because he couldn't stay and must return to his room at the rehab facility, far from home and garden.

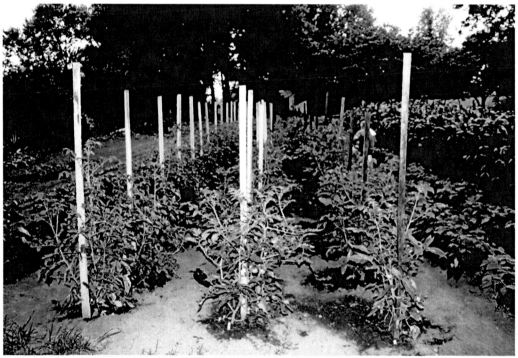

Staked Tomato Plants

Saturday, May 26, 2007

The garden was dry when I arrived at 10:00 this morning. We haven't had rain for many days and my last watering had disappeared into the parched soil. I stretched my hose pipe

(Nashville lingo for garden hose) to the garden and attached it to a long sprinkler hose that I had placed between the rows of corn. As I turned on the spigot, I could almost hear a sigh of relief from the thirsty corn plants.

My plan for the day was to run a sprinkler hose in the garden, which would allow me to do other tasks while a portion of the garden was being watered. I wanted to stake the remaining thirty one tomato plants, retie the ones I had already staked and tied, and weed a bit.

I checked in on Grandma and after assuring myself that she was fine, I started staking the tomatoes. The new poles that David had brought me were perfect and I drove them easily into the soil beside each plant. Tying the tomatoes was a little more trying because I had to squat for so long that it became hard for me to stand by the time I reached the thirty first stake.

I sat in the shade for a while and drank some water before moving the sprinkler hose and beginning the weeding. I found the day magnificent. The temperature was hovering around ninety degrees, but the humidity was low and a gentle breeze made the afternoon even more enjoyable.

As the day wore on, I found myself sitting more than weeding. The water falling on the plants was almost mesmerizing and my mind wandered to thoughts of Pop. He would have enjoyed sitting in this chair and watching me as I worked. He would have certainly been able to add some pointers to my efforts.

Sunday, May 27, 2007

I visited the garden this afternoon and took another set of pictures. I wanted to print them for Pop. Our tomato plants were covered in blooms and a couple of small tomatoes, and the beans had buds on them and were ready to flower.

I noticed that one of my bean plants was chopped off at the ground. After close inspection I determined that this was cutworm damage. I will research this on the internet and ask Pop what his preferred method of eradication is.

Cutworms or no cutworms, the garden has grown so much in the last week, and I hope when Pop sees the pictures he will be as proud and amazed as I am.

Monday, May 28, 2007

The Memorial Day weekend is past. Jason Barrett and I went to the garden at lunch and I showed him how to hook up the series of hoses I use to water the garden. Jason has volunteered to water the garden next week while I am on vacation. It is wonderful to have such friends and I will enjoy my time away knowing that the garden is in good hands. It was amazing to see that the beans had flowered since Sunday. The vitality of the garden has amazed me. I noticed that my Roma beans have white flowers on wispy runners, while the Contender beans have lavender flowers on short stalks.

I returned to the garden after work and planted two rows of Early Contender beans in the unused section at the rear of the garden. The squash will be planted when I return from vacation. I also hoed every row in the garden to remove fledgling weeds. I don't want to come home, following a week of rest and relaxation, to find the garden overrun with weeds.

While working along the rows with my hoe, I remembered our annual family vacations with Pop, Grandma, and our kids. Pop was always worried about his garden, and watched the weather nightly to see if Nashville was getting rain. By the end of the week he would often be frantic to get back home and water his garden. I never really appreciated his concern until now… Thank you Jason!

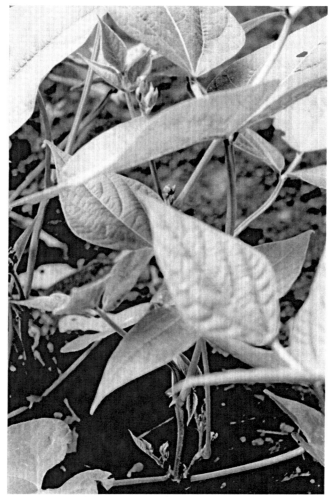
Early Contender Bean Plant

Wednesday, May 30, 2007

I dropped by at noon to check on Grandma and see if the cutworm had attacked another bean plant. I had read that the worm operated at night and would stay within three inches of the plant. My hope is that he has cut another stalk so that I can dig around and find him. This would be a more immediate and garden friendly resolution than spraying again. Alas, he has taken a rest and no new damage is found.

Friday, June 1, 2007

> *<u>Deuteronomy 11:13-14</u>: And it shall come to pass, if ye shall hearken diligently unto my commandments which I command you this day, to love the LORD your God, and to serve him with all your heart and with all your soul, That I will give the rain of your land in his due season, the first rain and the latter rain, that thou mayest gather in thy corn, and thy wine, and thine oil.*

Since I will be leaving tomorrow for vacation, I left work a couple of hours early so that I could water the garden before I left. There was no rain predicted until at least Sunday so this seemed to be a very good idea.

I rolled out my hoses and started watering the corn. As I moved between the rows and watered two rows on either side of me, I heard the rumble of thunder in the distance behind me. I continued along because the weather man had assured me that no rain was in the forecast.

I had nearly reached the far end of the row when I felt the first raindrop. It was large and created quite a wet spot on my shoulder. This was the kind of rain that teases you with a few large drops before suddenly ending. I continued watering. The raindrops started to come down more frequently and I glanced over my shoulder. I could see the rain moving towards me.

Quickly, I pulled the hose back and coiled it on the hanger at the end of the garden. By the time I reached the tool room (on a dead run) the rain was coming down buckets. I stood in the doorway and watched as the garden soaked up this unexpected, yet wonderful, rain.

As I watched the rain fall, I remembered the prayer that I had prayed when I started my venture. I had asked God to help me with this garden for Pop and to provide the rain and good growing conditions. I was immediately overcome with emotion as I wondered if God was showing me that he was upholding his end of this alliance. I thanked him out loud as I stood there with tears in my eyes, witnessing his greatness as the rain fell on a day that should have been dry.

Sunday, June 10, 2007

It was nine o'clock in the morning and I couldn't wait to see the garden. I walked into Pop and Grandma's house and yelled "Hello, is anyone home!"

Grandma met me before I could reach the kitchen door. She was glad that we were home and told me how much she had missed us. I told her that we had missed her as well and out of the corner of my eye I spotted the corn. In mid sentence I turned to stare out the window. The corn was head high and moving in the breeze. Grandma, seeing my surprise, immediately said that the garden was beautiful.

I excused myself and went to the garden. The corn was tall and healthy, the beans had pods on them that could be harvested, the tomato plants were heavy with green tomatoes, my newly planted rows of beans were breaking through the ground, and the melon vines were covered in blooms. Oh, and the weeds had fared well too.

I decided that my first order of business would be to tie the tomatoes again. They were drooping onto the ground. I would then run the tiller between the rows and hoe and weed the garden. There were several places that the tiller wouldn't be able to go. The rows of corn and beans had grown together, and the tomatoes were too close as well.

I retrieved the strings from the tool room and started tying up plants. This turned out to be quite a task. The plants had sprouted so much new growth that it took me half the day to make it through the three rows. Some of the stalks had split from the weight of the tomatoes, but I tied them up in the hope that they would continue to nourish the green gems that they supported. After reaching the final plant, I looked back over my work. Everything was in order again and the stakes were surrounded with lush green foliage.

I was almost beside myself as I pulled the tiller from the shed. I worked quickly around the melons, my peppers, and the new beans. I then went to the far end of the garden and moved between the rows of strawberries. The tiller made short work of the weeds that could be reached with it. I was glad that at least this much of the garden wouldn't need hoeing.

I retrieved the hoe from the tool room and started working the rows that I hadn't been able to reach with the tiller. The going was slow, but it felt good to be back in the garden. As I worked between the rows of head high corn, I thought back on my childhood when I would run between the rows on my grandfather's farm. I smiled to myself as I worked the row, dealing death to the pesky weeds.

By four o'clock the garden was looking like someone cared about it again. A great sense of satisfaction filled me as I looked out across the clean, orderly, rows. I could have stood there for hours, but Ann and I had plans to visit Pop at the Rehabilitation Home.

While we had been on vacation, it had been decided that Pop would return home on the thirteenth. He would need twenty four hour care, but he would be in his own home. As for me, I couldn't wait to wheel him to the garden in his wheelchair to see what we had accomplished together. The project that had been started for Pop was now about the two of us. I was developing the same attachment for this garden that Pop had cultivated so many years ago.

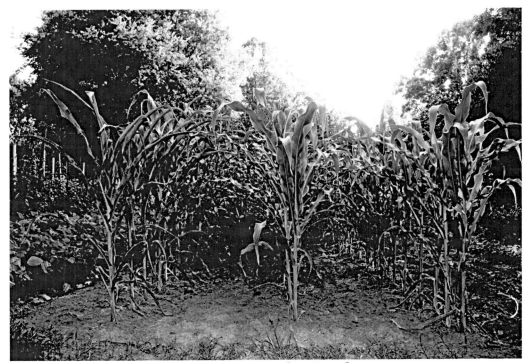
Sweet Corn in the Garden

Pop's Garden Gift

First Harvest

When the garden matures there comes a time of plenty, with plants hung heavy with vegetables. Canning and freezing are daily practices as the winter's store is laid up. All the while, the summer table is adorned with dishes made from fresh produce. The hours of planting and hoeing are replaced with the smells and tastes of summer.

Monday, June 11, 2007

I brought Jason Barrett to the garden at lunch to give me a quick lesson on which beans were ready to harvest. With Pop still at the Rehab Home, I needed some on-site help. Jason gave me his rule of thumb… "If they are as big around as a pencil and about six inches long, they're ready." He reinforced the rule by showing me several examples. We decided that the Early Contenders were ready for their first pick, but the Roma IIs were still a couple of days away.

I decided to run home after work and change clothes before returning to pick the first real harvest from the garden. I brought a white five gallon bucket to sit on and a basket for the beans. By planting the beans in half rows, I was able to set the bucket between the rows and pick from either side of me without having to move all the way down a single row.

I gently moved and lifted the thick cover of leaves to reveal the bean pods as I worked my way along. Not all of the beans had matured at once, so there would be another picking in a few days. By the time I reached the end of the Contender beans, I had filled half of a gallon basket with beautiful pencil sized beans. The Roma II beans weren't ready to be picked yet, so I took my harvest and went to the patio.

I placed the basket of beans beside me on one side and an open grocery bag on the other. Working quickly, I pinched off the end of each pod and then snapped it into pieces about an inch long; placing the pieces in the grocery bag. By the time I had snapped all of the beans, I had filled the grocery bag with enough beans to make several meals.

Proudly, I took the beans into the house and presented them to Grandma. She heaped praise on them as she informed me that they would be cooked for Pop's homecoming. "He loves fresh beans" she said. I smiled and shook my head in agreement. The feeling was wonderful and I was glad that Pop would be home just in time to taste the first proceeds from the garden.

<u>Wednesday, June 13, 2007</u>

Today was a very special day. Pop was being released from the Rehab Facility and would be returning to Wilhugh Place. David and Susanne Young had made arrangements for around the clock care, and Don Young would bring him home.

Pop had reached the point where Ann and Grandma couldn't care for him alone. He needed to be lifted, and neither of them was capable of doing that. It was hard on the family to see him in such a diminished state. He could shuffle for short distances with his walker, but for all intents and purposes, he was confined to a wheel chair.

I left work, changed clothes, and went to the garden. We haven't had rain this week and I needed to water. I especially didn't want Pop to see the garden wilted or starving for water.

After hooking up the hoses, I started watering the tomato plants. I was amazed that they had grown to the point that I would need to tie them up again. How could a plant grow this much without rain?

I walked along watering the three rows of tomatoes and one of my new rows of beans. While stretching to water the far row of tomatoes, I noticed that my Roma Beans needed to be picked. I watered further down the row and noticed that the Contenders were loaded with beans as well. It amazed me that the Contenders were ready to be picked again. I had just picked them two days ago… My watering would have to wait. If I didn't pick beans tonight, they would get too big and become tough.

Just as I was finishing the last tomato plants, I saw Holly and Jane Ann walking up to the garden. Jane Ann was excited to see me in the garden and called for me to hold her. I remembered my children calling to Pop in this same garden and the continuity of the moment was not lost on me.

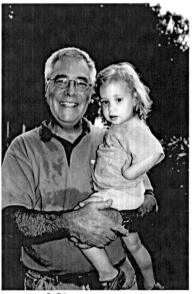

Holding Jane Ann

I was holding Jane Ann when Ann walked up to the garden with the camera. It had been a while since she saw the garden and she was amazed. Jane Ann wanted her "Mimi" to hold her so I took the opportunity to begin picking beans. As I worked my way down the rows, Ann took pictures of the garden and on occasion asked me to turn around so that she could see my face in her view finder. The afternoon had become a family outing and the memories of past gatherings around the garden flooded back.

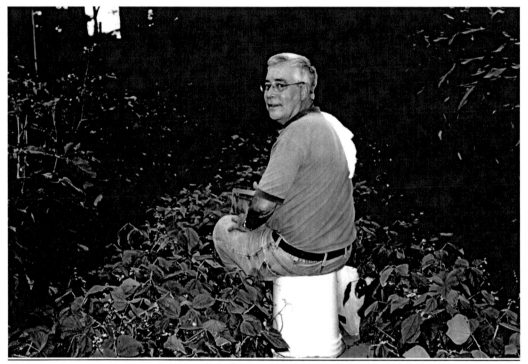
Picking Beans

Soon I was alone again in the garden. I picked frantically trying to reach the end of the rows before darkness fell, but much to my dismay, I wasn't able to do this. I finished my picking in the dark. It was interesting that I was able to see the Roma beans against the darker leaves of the plant. I could then feel them with my hand and determine if they were ready to be picked. I know that I missed many, but at the end of the row I had a full five gallon bucket of beans.

It was nine thirty when I finished putting up my things and walked into the house. Pop had arrived home while I was in the garden and was eating a big piece of chocolate cake. It was evident that he was glad to be back at home.

I held the beans where Pop could see them and he remarked on their size and beauty. He asked me several questions about the rest of the garden and I promised to come over after work tomorrow and take him to the garden. I told him that I would push him up there in his wheelchair to which he responded that he could make it with his walker. I knew that this would be impossible for him, so I told him that it would be less tiring if he would let me take him in the wheelchair. He agreed, but I knew that we would have this conversation again tomorrow evening. I was glad to have my mentor at home once again, and despite his much weakened state, I had the feeling that things were better now. It is hard to explain why I felt this way because I knew that he could never return to the garden unassisted again.

Pop's Garden Gift

Final Harvest

Final harvest usually comes in the early winter and with both sadness, and a little relief as well, thoughts turn toward preparing the ground for the cold days ahead. Some years however, the gardening season can be cut short by drought, blight, or some other natural disaster. In the case of my garden with Pop, such a natural disaster occurred, and winter came early to our garden.

Thursday, June 14, 2007

Pop had an especially bad evening last night. He suffered a severe case of delirium and is remarkably weaker than he has been. I decided to forego any work in the garden today.

Saturday, June 16, 2007

I arrived at Pop's house about nine o'clock in the morning. I thought about watering the garden, but decided to just pick the beans instead. Pop's health was so poor that I felt a bit of depression. As a result, I was having a hard time separating my feelings for the garden from those I had for him.

I started picking beans and lost myself in the job. It was a hot morning, but the sweat seemed to purify my spirit as I moved down the rows plucking beautiful beans from their leafy green homes. The prolific plants seemed to produce more beans with each harvest and by the time I had reached the end of my task, I had accumulated nearly eight gallons of beans. This was the largest amount I had picked yet.

When I had put most of the beans in my car, I took a basket of the Early Contenders into the house and showed them to Pop. Without picking his head up from the chair cushion, he turned slowly to see the beans. A smile came on his face and he said "they are beautiful, how many tomatoes are on the vines?' I responded that the vines were covered, but that the drought was keeping them smaller than we would have hoped. He closed his eyes and continued to talk. "Are there any cantaloupes on the vines?" I said that they were covered in blooms, but no melons yet. Pop began to speak again, but fell asleep in mid sentence. I gently rubbed his arm and whispered that I would see him tomorrow.

Sunday, June 17, 2007

Ann and I visited Pop around noon. It was Father's Day and Ann wanted to take him a box of his favorite chocolate. When we walked into the house, Pop greeted Ann immediately. He seemed to have regained some of his strength. Pop asked if Ann could help the nurse bathe him and also asked if I would give him a shave. We both agreed.

We helped him into the shower and Ann gently bathed him and washed his hair. Once clean, dried, and dressed, I took his razor from the medicine cabinet and lathered his face. I asked him if he could remember the first thing he said to me when we met. He responded "yes." I recounted the story of him asking me if I had lost my razor and we all laughed. He grew solemn and said "giving up my daughter was the hardest thing I ever did." I remarked that he probably never envisioned that same bearded young man shaving him thirty some years later and he responded "No." As if lost in a thought he said "We've had a wonderful life haven't we?" Ann and I responded "Yes we have."

Following the bath, Pop returned to his favorite chair. Ann asked him if he would like to go to the garden this evening and he said that he would, but didn't know if he could make it. She explained that our son Chris would be here and that between Chris and me we would put him in his wheelchair and push him up to the garden. Grandma had asked us to come for dinner this evening and we set the time for five o'clock. I left a gallon bag of washed and snapped beans with Grandma for our evening meal.

We returned at five and with Chris's help placed Pop in his wheelchair. The ride across the back yard was a bit bumpy and I had to stop occasionally and help him sit upright in the chair. This was a ride that I had doubted that Pop would ever make again.

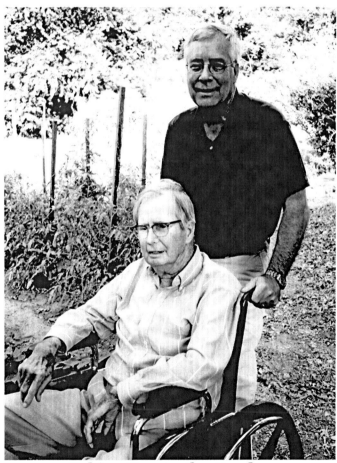

Taking Pop to the Garden

Soon we were entering the garden. Pop was amazed at the growth and wanted to see everything. He gave me instructions as we went from row to row. Finally we passed the tomatoes and he was able to see the hills of melons. "They look great!" he said with a smile on his face. "Do they have any melons yet?" I said no, but they were covered in blooms as he could see. Ann snapped pictures as we went, and I was glad that she was recording this moment. It was special for Pop, and also for each of us there.

My only regret regarding the trip to the garden was that the ninety five degree heat and drought had caused the plants to droop down during the day. It always looks better in the mornings and I especially wanted the garden to look good upon Pop's return.

<u>Wednesday, June 20, 2007</u>

After two days of rain showers, I returned to the garden to pick beans. The amount of growth was astonishing! The corn was now towering over my head and was crowned with tassels. I looked closely at the cantaloupe vines and in addition to the flowers, they had several melons on them. The largest was approximately the size of a softball. As for the new rows of beans I had planted, they were doubled in size.

I retrieved my five gallon bucket and set it between the original rows of beans as a seat. I started picking beans at about six thirty and finished at nine o'clock. It had been four days since I picked, and the beans were plentiful and large. By the end of the rows, I had nearly ten gallons of beans. This was my largest single picking yet.

After putting the beans in my car, I went in to say goodbye to Grandma and Pop. They were finishing their Wednesday evening dinner with Don and Christine Young and offered me some of Don's birthday cake. The offer was too good to resist and I had a piece.

While eating my cake, I informed Pop that we had cantaloupes in the garden. He was excited at the prospect and quizzed me regarding size and quantity. We went on to discuss the amount of growth and the positive effect the rain had on our efforts. Finishing my dessert, I said my goodbyes and leaned down to tell Pop that I would bring some beans over in the morning. He took my hand and held it. "Thank you for all you are doing" he said and continued to hold my hand. His grip was weak, but loving. We shared something that had taken our relationship to a special level. I could have held his hand forever. In a near whisper I said "I'll see you in the morning" and walked quietly from the house.

Saturday, June 23, 2007

I have been to Pop and Grandma's several times over the past days, but it wasn't to garden. Pop's health has deteriorated significantly and the family has been gathering around him. We received a call early this morning from my daughter Mariah who informed us that Pop was much worse. If we wanted to see him, we should come right away.

By the time Ann and I arrived at Pop's, he had recovered from his episode, but he was still semi coherent and he was unable to answer questions that took more than a moment to think about. His breathing was labored and slow, but this was consistent with his state over the past few days so I left Ann with him and headed to the garden to pick beans.

The garden was my retreat and a place I could feel close to Pop without watching his struggle. I picked a few gallons of beans, between silent prayers, and surveyed the garden. The tomato plants were covered in green tomatoes, the cantaloupes vines now contained several new cantaloupes, the watermelon plants had new little watermelons extending from the vegetation and the corn stalks had small ears of corn protruding from them.

When I returned to the house, Pop's eyes were closed. I sat on the couch beside him and he immediately opened them and looked at me. I told him that we had some nice cantaloupes and that his watermelon vines were now sporting beautiful little melons that looked like miniature versions of the full grown fruit. He smiled and asked me about the tomatoes but, as I was responding, his eyes closed once again.

After visiting with Grandma, Ann and I returned home to perform our weekend chores and feed the boys. The day was busy, but by early afternoon the phone rang again and Ann's brother Don summoned us back to Pop's side. He had regressed once again and Don was afraid he might not make nightfall.

Pop's condition, although bad, seemed stable and he continued to show great courage and a will to live. His breathing had slowed to a breath every ten or fifteen seconds and each would come with great difficulty. We finally left him in the care of his nurse and went home at one o'clock in the morning.

<u>Monday, June 25, 2007</u>

Mariah stopped by Pop's on her way to work this morning and found him sitting in his wheelchair reading the morning paper. He was coherent and able to speak. She didn't notice the labored breathing that was so disturbing over the weekend. I thanked God for the recovery, but knew that this cycle would be repeated again as his heart continued to weaken.

Ann and I visited Doctor Van Devender and discussed the situation with him. We made arrangements for Hospice care to begin tomorrow. The situation was grave and time was short. Pop was complaining of constant pain and deserved relief.

I asked God to let him taste his tomatoes and melons before he called him home. It had rained overnight and there were showers predicted for every day this week. Was God providing for the garden in answer to my prayer before I had even voiced the words?

Wednesday, June 27, 2007

It has been another bad day for Pop's health. The family has gathered around him and he is slipping away. Hospice delivered a hospital bed yesterday and for the most part he lays there with his eyes closed, breathing inconsistently; one or two breaths per minute. I stood beside him and held his hand for a long while and told him that I loved him. He squeezed my hand but never opened his eyes.

Ann has found a strength that I have never seen in her as she tends to her father's needs. She is grieving and I wish that I could take that away, but her love is too strong for that. She needs to travel this road with him.

I walked up to the garden to clear my thoughts and found that a deer had visited the night before. It had wandered up and down the rows of vegetables. This is surprising because the garden is in a subdivision of Metropolitan Nashville. Several of the tomato plants had fallen, but a brief summer storm yesterday evening may have been to blame. I walked back down to the house and announced my finding to Ann as she comforted Pop. He opened his eyes and looked at me as I spoke.

Even in his diminished state, Pop reacts to news of the garden. David asked him if the deer might eat the cantaloupes and in a raspy voice he responded "yes," before slipping back into his sleeplike state.

Previously, in my grief, I had fleetingly considered plowing the garden under, but that would never be something I could do. It would be akin to giving up a piece of Pop and I wanted to hang onto every memory we had made together in our garden on Wilhugh Place. Pop would always be alive in that soil and in the plants that grew there. I knew that this was one place we could always feel close to him.

Thursday, June 28, 2007

Yesterday afternoon I visited Dr. Van Devender for my annual physical. Before the exam he took me to his office and closed the door. I sat in a chair facing his desk and he asked me about Mr. Young (Pop). "Is he dying?" I thought the question odd, but responded "yes, he is." We then talked about the garden and what Pop and I had planted. After I listed all of our plants, he asked me another odd question. "Did you plant any cotton?" I chuckled and replied "No." (Even a novice such as me knew that cotton couldn't be eaten.) He went on to tell me that he planted cotton seeds in a pot each year.

I was sitting in Centennial Medical Center's Imaging Lab this morning waiting to have an ultrasound taken of my thyroid gland. Dr. Van Devender had felt a lump and scheduled me for a follow up image. As I thought back to my visit with him and the seemingly odd questions he had asked me, it suddenly became clear why he had asked them.

The first question had been "Is he dying?" I now realized that he was gauging my acceptance of the fact that Pop was indeed dying. He was looking for an indication of my progress in dealing with this inevitability. He wanted to know how I was handling this life changing event… He already knew that Pop was dying.

The second question had been "Did you plant any cotton?" I knew that Dr. Van Devender was from Mississippi, but what I missed was that the cotton plant was a link to his home and to memories he held dear. I suddenly realized that I had indeed planted "cotton," it was our tomatoes, our cantaloupes, and our watermelons; the plants Pop loved best. I sat there and pondered a deeper question. Would I plant MY cotton every year? Would I keep my memories alive in the same way that Karl did his?

Now I knew why Pop had recommended Dr. Van Devender to Ann and me when we were looking for a family physician. He had seen in him a doctor who treated more than just your body. He saw a man who understood the importance of planting cotton.

Friday, June 29, 2007

Mid afternoon Ann called me at work with the urgent news that Pop's death was imminent. I quickly shut down my office and drove to Pop and Grandma's. He was struggling to stay with us and every breath was a challenge. I leaned over and took his hand to tell him I was there and loved him. There was no response.

The family gathered. Family was the most important part of Pop's life and they were there beside him; Children, Grandchildren, Great Grandchildren, Sisters, and best of all, Grandma.

The afternoon wore on into early evening and I needed to find a quiet place to ease my grief. I walked up to the garden and looked at the tomato plants that were still lying where the storm had knocked them over. I was lost.

Instinctively, I picked up my five gallon bucket and started picking beans. It was work that took me to an easier time and was comforting. I was picking along when I heard my son Chris call me from the edge of the garden. "Can I help dad?"

I told Chris that the tomatoes needed to be tied up, but that I would need to show him how. "I already know how dad" he responded. "Pop showed me how when I worked in the garden with him." I had forgotten that when Chris was a boy, Pop would ask for him to come over to help in the yard. I said, "That will be great; the strings are in the tool room."

We worked along together picking beans, tying tomatoes, and remembering the good times we shared in the garden with Pop. By dark Chris had tied up half the tomatoes and I had picked two large baskets of beans. The garden was comforting us.

When we walked back to the house I remembered Pop's joy in sharing the bounty of his garden. Ann met me on the patio and I showed her the beans. I asked her to offer them to Pop's sisters, Eunice and Ruby… They were happy to have them and I could almost see Pop smiling. Gifts continued to flow from the garden.

<u>Saturday, June 30, 2007</u>

At Two Forty in the morning the phone rang. Joe Young told me that Pop was gone and that Ann was having a rough time. I told him that I would be there momentarily, and hung up the receiver. Earlier that night I had returned home to be with the boys. Ann and her brothers remained behind to be with their father.

I pulled into the dark driveway and turned off the car. My heart was breaking as I walked up the wheelchair ramp to the door. Pop was lying in his hospital bed and I couldn't help but touch him with a gentle hand. He had suffered so mightily. I held Ann and comforted her as she hugged me and wept. We were heart broken.

Later in the morning, David and I were standing beside Pop's vacant hospital bed talking when I noticed a beautiful doe deer standing in the front yard. We called Grandma and watched until the doe became alarmed and ran to safety through a neighbor's yard.

Tuesday, July 3, 2007

After Two days of visitation with family and friends, we buried Pop. Our tears found new depths and hearts ached. Pastors L.H. Hardwick and Dan Scott delivered wonderful messages and remembrances of his life and the impact he had on his church and church family. He had transformed the church grounds into a garden paradise. Following the burial, Ann and I went to Pop and Grandma's house to join the rest of the family there. We spent time together eating and remembering Pop.

After visiting for a while, I wandered off to the garden. It was hard to see his folding chair sitting against the fence, but I needed to be in this place that he loved. I walked to the rows of tomatoes and saw a large ripe tomato. I was amazed that it chose this day to ripen. I picked it and immediately saw another… and another. I went to the house and found a basket. Returning to the garden, I filled the basket with large ripe tomatoes. Tears filled my eyes; I had wanted Pop to see our first tomatoes.

As I picked, I knew what needed to be done. Pop would have wanted Dan Scott and Karl Van Devender to receive a basket of his vine ripe tomatoes. I would be Pop's emissary, his delivery boy, for this last gift of love and respect.

I felt the honor associated with my position. This delivery would complete our garden and honor his memory in a very special way… his way.

Friday, July 6, 2007

I returned to the garden to tie up the remaining tomato plants. My son Chris joined me there and we lifted and tied the vines. Together we picked another full basket of beautiful tomatoes. We worked, and talked of Pop. It was a wonderful day of remembrance. It reaffirmed the closeness of family that Pop found so important. This garden was all about family and, over the years, every member of the family had worked it.

Monday, July 9, 2007

Jason Barrett agreed to look at my corn during lunch. Without my mentor, I was at a loss as to when I should pick. We determined that the Silver Queen corn was ready for picking today. Moving to the back of the garden Jason instructed me on what to look for to determine when the cantaloupes would be ready. They were full size, but hadn't fully ripened yet.

I arrived at the garden late in the afternoon and, with a five gallon bucket in hand, began picking ears of corn. I emptied the bucket twice before reaching the end of the rows. My first pick yielded eighty six perfectly formed ears. Pop would have been proud, and there were many more ears that would be ready in the next few days.

The tomatoes continue to produce and another full basket of red beauties was delivered to Ann. She will use them to can chili sauce and season it with tears for her father; tears of love.

Thursday, July 12, 2007

I took a basket full of beautiful red tomatoes to Dr. Karl Van Devender along with a note explaining that they were a gift from Mr. Young's garden. Karl would need no reminder of their significance.

Friday, July 13, 2007

> *Numbers 18:12: All the best of the oil, and all the best of the wine, and of the wheat, the firstfruits of them which they shall offer unto the LORD, them have I given thee.*

Today I completed the journey that Pop and I had begun so many months ago; I delivered a large basket of tomatoes, which I had set aside, to Pastor Dan Scott at Christ Church. Dan always commanded a special place in Pop's heart.

Our garden odyssey had started as a gift and it was only fitting that it should end in the same way. This is how Pop would have wanted it. This is how I had dreamed it.

Pop's Garden Gift

Planting Cotton

The garden continues to yield vegetables by the basket full. I work it and think of Pop and our days of planning, preparation, planting, and harvest. When autumn comes there will be turnip greens and other fall produce. Although the plants will grow, yield their fruit, and die, I know that Pop will always be found here in this garden.

Throughout the days when he was receiving hospice care, each of his children would bring their families to this garden and tell them of Pop's love for gardening. It drew them here without fail; it was his legacy. Sometimes they would just stand and look, at other times they would wipe tears from their eyes, but always they would remember.

Last fall I started this garden as a gift to Pop. I thought that my efforts would make him happy and let him relive the glorious spectacle that was his garden. Maybe there was truth in this, but I came to realize that much different gifts had been given. This garden had become Pop's gift to me, and much more.

Pop had received my offering and used it to teach me about life, about giving, about family, about love, and about God. He had taken my gift and done with it what he always seemed to do; he had improved on it and given it back to me.

As I watched his children and grandchildren come to the garden, I realized that this gift had also been extended to them. It was a living growing extension of him. He was lying in the grasp of death, but his essence was here and he was giving them this act of love and charity as his parting gift.

I only hope that Pop's children, grandchildren, and great grandchildren, fully understand that this garden is precious. It is a memory that binds our family together; a gift of love that we can share as we grow old. With God's grace, perhaps we can leave gardens for our own children to plant in remembrance of us.

Doctor Karl Van Devender had once asked me if I planted Cotton, and I didn't know how to respond. Today I know the meaning and importance of planting cotton and am a better man for it. I also witnessed first hand how much God could stuff into a small seed, and I praise him for that. Pop had shown me that even the smallest of God's works is a miracle.

> *Genesis 2:8: And the LORD God planted a garden eastward in Eden; and there he put the man whom he had formed.*

There are evenings in the garden when the wind falls still and the sun sits low in the western sky that my mind is set free to wander. As the clouds swirl in hues of orange and lavender, I dwell on thoughts of heaven and God. In moments such as this I see, in my mind's eye, a gardener working the soil to produce an offering suitable for his Lord. I can't imagine a more magnificent vision in heaven than the garden our LORD God planted eastward in Eden for the man he had formed.

If indeed there is a garden in heaven, then I am certain that this is where Pop awaits us.

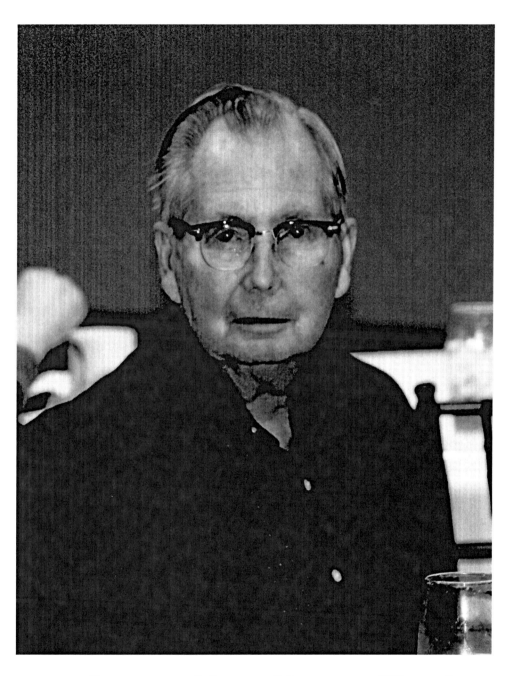

James Alton Young (Pop)

Printed in the United States
107572LV00003B/275-302/P